What People are Saying about **Your Best Body Ever**

Joanna's review...

"I have turned some bad habits into good habit especially around eating and taking the time to appreciate the world. My endurance levels have improved. Making a list of what you are grateful for has really focused my mind and made me stop and think. Suddenly things didn't seem so bad."

Theresa's review...

"I've lost half a stone in the past 6 months and my body shape has changed. I am now toned in my middle, bum and thighs. My arms are toned too. I'm going to have to buy some new clothes as all my clothes feel too big and with my new shape and don't fit properly. The nourishing mind questions have bought about a special awareness and appreciation of life. I was feeling low after the passing of my late husband a year ago but I am now so much more positive and confident. My family have noticed and enjoying a more positive and happier me."

Sallie's review...

"I was worried I'd lose strength and fitness if I didn't start doing something about it! In just a few months, I'm stronger and more toned. I've been able to strengthen and make more mobile my weak shoulder."

Jonathan's review...

"During the last 10 months I've lost 2 stone, my asthma has improved tremendously and I am so much fitter. I have completely changed my eating habits and am convinced the combination of great daily physical and mental fitness habits coupled with good nutrition has made the difference. When I look back at my photos, I can see what a 'unit' I used to be!"

Your Best Body Ever

ANNA SCANLAN

Editor: Corinne L. Casazza
corinnecasazza@gmail.com

Cover & Book Design: Anne Karklins
annekarklins@gmail.com

ISBN 13: 978-1-989161-53-1
ISBN 10: 1989161537

Hasmark
PUBLISHING

Dedication

For my ray of positive sunshine teacher family spanning back several generations. They've been so skilled at instilling the excitement of learning, improving and advancing. Particularly my dear mum Christine always exuding such belief and support with words of 'you can do it' ringing in my ears.

The sun goes up and the sun goes down with certainty.
The laws of the universe have the same certainty.
Define your focus and give full attention to your dreams and heart's desires and your greater life is yours for the taking.

– Anna Scanlan

Acknowledgements

I am so happy and grateful for the inspirational teachers, coaches and experts I have been blessed to have in my life. True professionals, brilliant mentors, always giving encouragement with a knowing, calm belief in me.

Held in such high regard we have:

John Beer – Personal Coach for Olympic Games in Gymnastics & Trampolining. Sports psychology expert. National Champion.

Mike Hammond – Paralympic Winter Olympic Competitor and top level expert Ski Instructor/Coach/Trainer of Trainers. Sports phycology expert, working on your inner game.

Bob Proctor – Legend in developing human potential with the mind.

Peggy McCall – *New York Times* Best Selling Author. Captivating and awe-inspiring expert public speaker. Phenomenal life/business coach and mentor. Expert in transformative personal development. An innovative and inspiring entrepreneur developer.

Mary Morrissey – Life Mastery Mentor in health, relationships, vocation and time/money freedom.

Lucy Johnson – Business School in Health, Fitness and Wellness. Clever techniques to grow your business and help more clients. Developing confidence with mindset.

Tony Robbins – World renowned life coach in awakening potential.

Oprah Winfrey – Admire you greatly and love your take on life. Such an inspiration. You really can be the person you want to be and not let conditions and circumstance hold you back.

Thank you for imparting such invaluable knowledge, adding fuel to my passions and accelerating my advancement towards my life purpose, dreams, wants and desires. I wouldn't be the person I am today without your help and inspiration.

It certainly highlights; we all need mentors, coaches, and similar mindset groups to advance in the direction we want to go. Enjoying a more healthy, vibrant, joyful, fit and abundant life really is there for the taking especially and essentially from the right experts and mentors around us.

www.yourbestbodyever.com

Note from Author

Welcome to this little body and mind nourishing book. You must be holding this book for a good reason. You're sensing a burning desire for change welling up inside you. You're ready to embark on the most important mission of your life, looking after your magnificent body and mind. You've recognized that there is a mind body connection, and you're ready to make positive changes. Body care and mind care are equally important and require your full, undivided and equal attention.

You've attracted this book into your hands and can now discover the secrets of melting away the bad habits and make good habits the new normal.

You'll discover ways of looking after yourself made super uncomplicated in *Your Best Body Ever*. You'll get an easy-to- follow 5 point daily plan that makes healthy choices second nature.

This is an all-around, holistic solution, working on your healthy body and healthy mind for happiness, longevity, well-living, fitness and great health. Plus, the happier you are the less likely you'll want to comfort eat.

Imagine if every year you were getting younger? I certainly can't guarantee eternal youth, but you'd be surprised with a bit of care and attention you really can transform yourself and make the most of what you've got.

Plus, why not enjoy the journey, have fun and glee as you nourish and nurture your magnificent physical body and change your thinking mind for a greater life?

Table of Contents

Part 1 Your Pre-plan Work

Aperitif – Introduction   19

Food for thought   21

Three Clients, their stories   21

Raise a Toast – Decision   23

Chatter – Habitual beings   23

Spice up your life – Get clear on your goal   23

Dream for a bit   25

Part II The Five Point Daily Plan

Easy as 1, 2, 3, 4, 5   27

Your 5 point daily plan   27

Cheers for Gratitude   27

Nature for wellbeing – marvel the beauty whilst walking   28

Best body Fuel – Balanced Meals   28

Nourishing Mind Questions – Happiness boosters   31

Best Body – 5 components of fitness   33

Habit re-programming   49

Making the most of your Five Point Daily Plan   49

Final thoughts   53

Part III The Recipes

LEEK AND SWEET POTATO SOUP (Vegetarian & Vegan)   55

MILD CURRIED CHICKPEA & VEGETABLE SOUP (Vegetarian & Vegan)   56

SPICED CARROT & LENTIL SOUP (Vegetarian & Vegan)   57

TOMATO & ROSEMARY SOUP (Vegetarian & Vegan)   58

CELERY SOUP (Vegetarian & Vegan)   59

CARROT AND GINGER SOUP (Vegetarian & Vegan)   60

CHICKEN, SPRING PEAS AND ASPARAGUS QUINOA   61

TURKEY & GARLIC ROASTED VEGETABLES   62

QUINOA SALAD WITH AVOCADO, TOMATO, PARSLEY & PINE NUTS (Vegetarian & Vegan)   63

BUCKWHEAT PATTIES (BALLS) (Vegetarian & Vegan)   64

ROASTED SPICY PARSNIP (Vegetarian & Vegan)   65

LIME CHILI STIR FRY (Vegetarian & Vegan)   66

CHICKPEA PATTIES WITH TOMATO, CUCUMBER & MINT SALAD (Vegetarian & Vegan)   67

ROAST CHICKEN – NUT & ONION   68

STEAMED SALMON & HUMMUS   69

QUINOA & CAJUN CHICKEN   70

CRAB STEW   72

COURGETTE HUMMUS (Vegetarian & Vegan)   73

GRILLED/GRIDDLE CHINESE CHICKEN   74

COD CEVICHE   75

BEAN SPOUT & RED CABBAGE SALAD (Vegetarian & Vegan)   76

WARM CHICKEN SALAD   77

SPICY VEGGIE BURGERS (Vegetarian)   78

SALAD NICOISE   79

SCALLOPS   80

FISH POTATO BAKE   81

BEETROOT SALAD (Vegetarian & Vegan)   82

PRAWN HOTPOT   83

GRIDDLED AUBERGINE (Vegetarian & Vegan)   84

AVOCADO & TOFU DIP (Vegetarian & Vegan)   85

SALMON ASPARAGUS PARCELS   86

SPICY TUNA IN TOMATO SAUCE   87

CHILLI LIME DRESSING (Vegetarian & Vegan)   88

CITRUS DRESSING (Vegetarian & Vegan)   89

THOUSAND ISLAND DRESSING   90

HOMEMADE MAYONNAISE   91

BALSAMIC MARINADE (Vegetarian & Vegan)   92

Reference   93

Foreword

By Peggy McColl

Have you ever longed to be healthy, have lots of energy, and be comfortable with your life? Are you struggling for change or wanting to build new habits? Are you living your best life?

We all want to live a healthy lifestyle; and most of us have lifestyle habits we would like to change. Imagine a time not too far from now... where you feel great and have more energy than ever before. Where you are in control of your health and your life. Wouldn't it be nice for someone to give you a prescription for wellness, AND even the steps to implement it?

If you've been waiting for a push to create your best life, the book in your hands is about making the "when" happen "now." *Your Best Body Ever* provides you with the road map and tools to nourish your body and mind. It incorporates physical and mental fitness through nutrition and fitness; and propels you toward a greater, happier and more enriched life.

Lifestyle coach Anna Scanlan takes you on a journey that reveals how her holistic 5 point daily plan can result in dynamic and lasting change. This generous, determined, get-it-done kind of lady has created a step-by-step formula to help individuals create new healthy habits in order to help them look younger and feel younger, healthier and happier.

How will you achieve extraordinary results in every area of your life?

A healthy lifestyle is much more than a simple change in a workout routine or short-term diet. Being healthy is a way of life. This book will teach you how to form positive habits such as thinking positively and feeling gratitude at all times, and will improve your health in many ways.

Your Best Body Ever takes a three-pronged approach to a healthy lifestyle, covering nutrition, exercise, and mindset, and showing how each is interconnected and plays its own important role in overall health. Anna's Five Point Daily Plan will lead you to a healthier, more energetic, and more productive life – helping you to live the life you want, not just the one you have.

Each stage of the Five Point Daily Plan is comprehensively explained, with action items, tools, and resources to enable you to follow through and effect change in your life. The five stages are:

1. Cheers – Gratitude
2. Nature for Well-being
3. Best body fuel – balanced meals
4. Nourishing Mind Questions - Happiness boosters
5. Best Body 5 Components of Fitness Routines

The book also includes stories of Anna's clients, which many of us can relate to, and covers changing and forming new habits. It also covers nutrition, from the best foods to eat (carbs, proteins, fats) to portion sizes to providing several mouth-watering healthy recipes.

From there Anna moves into the realm of physical activity, providing examples of workout routines and outlining the basic types of exercises with their proper forms. And Anna understands that putting into practice the nutrition and exercise techniques recommended in the book takes motivation and dedication, which is where the "healthy mind" comes into play.

Your Best Body Ever includes a section focused on setting attainable goals that you can achieve and feel great about, thereby building confidence internally, giving you the tools necessary to integrate healthy eating and exercise habits into your daily life.

Utilize the Power of Habit to Make Positive Changes in Your Life

There is no shortcut to great health or performance, but *Your Best Body Ever* gives you the knowledge and tools you need to make lifestyle changes that will provide lifelong habits that will empower you to live a healthier lifestyle, to lose weight, or just be the best version of yourself so you can live your best life in your best body ever!

You and you alone will have to put in all of the physical and mental work required to transform. If you are doing it correctly, then it will be hard work over time that will see you to your goals… much like anything else in life.

I have read many books in the self-help field throughout my life; but I have to say Anna's book is on top of my list. It is clear, concise, challenging, and offers an opportunity to change ourselves to live a happy and meaningful life.

It is easy to get caught up in the diets and programs that are offered everywhere we look, but Anna reminds readers, that real change starts when one establishes habits, and slowly works at them over time. She leads you toward a life of growth and contribution that will enable you to become the happiest, healthiest, and most fulfilled version of yourself – and inspire you to help others do the same.

As Lao Tzu said, "*The journey of a 1000 miles begins with one step.*" The author has provided you with the first step… the rest are yours if you want it!

Peggy McColl, *New York Times* Best-Selling Author of *Your Destiny Switch*

http://PeggyMcColl.com

Preface

I believe the number one priority for the human race is physical and mental fitness with healthy living for a greater life. I believe anything is possible at any age. With the right application of your efforts it's possible to look younger, feel younger and take up activities thought not suitable in a certain age bracket! It doesn't take that much effort if you know what to do, decide you're going to do it and place daily importance on it.

Yes, I'm 50 years young! I feel top of the world and better than ever. I have so much energy. I take daily care of my physical and mental fitness and make carefully selected meal choices.

My background is an expert consultant, trainer and encourager of people in respect of fitness, nutrition, personal development and use of the mind for a great life. I've worked with thousands of people to help bring the best out of themselves and imprint some decent, well-living habits for long term success. Helping you to look younger, feel younger, boost confidence, have more energy, great health and living a more enriched life.

I come from a family of school teachers and am grateful for lesson plans and discussions on teaching as it's helped me to always look for ingenious ways of getting a point across in an understandable, easily converted way so it sticks and is forever of benefit. I love helping people help themselves and stay on the right track. I've always been interested in peak living with knowing the right ways to exercise, eat and think, living well and feeling young into forever. I've invested thousands of dollars in personal development courses with a strong emphasis on how we think to make a difference.

Working on self, to some seems self-indulgent, to me it's absolutely essential for everyone and an aid to making the most of your precious time on this awesome planet. I'm all about making the most of yourself to make the most of your life. To not only benefit you, but also all your loved ones and people around you. I'm sending positive thoughts and love to you and all in the world to make it a better place for all.

I certainly don't take good health for granted. I've been lucky enough to enjoy it most of my life. Ten years ago, I discovered that clearly there was a mind body connection with your thinking affecting your health. After the death of my son's father from lung cancer at just 39, I was so shocked and ill that I lost my voice.

I just couldn't speak for nine months. During that time, I saw lots of specialists: voice coach, hypnotherapist, cranial osteopath, physiotherapist and councillors. There was so much tension in the voice box area of my neck and I still couldn't speak. I was getting more and more upset, feeling anxious and worried this would be a permanent condition.

Trying to discover what caused this and how to cure it was quite a task. I wondered if a Botox injection in my neck would loosen my neck muscles so I could speak. The idea was confirmed by a woman I met at a yoga class who had a continuous twitch on the side of her face and eye. She had three monthly Botox injections to stop the twitch. A light bulb went off in my head. I went to see the doctor and discovered it was a viable treatment. The doctor referred me to the hospital, yes there were a few risks but what was the worst that could happen?

During the three weeks leading up to the hospital appointment all I could think about was how I was going to be able to speak again and all the things I could to do with a voice. My dear mum (Christine) drove me as I wasn't supposed to drive myself back. I had the initial consultation then was issued the front facing gown with just the underpants (I was thinking, was this really necessary for just my neck?) While lying on the hospital bed waiting for my injection, I kept repeating in my mind that the Botox would cure me and that I would be able to speak again. Over and over again thinking positive thoughts and visualising success.

Two hours passed and the consultant returned only to apologise saying they didn't have the correct Botox and I'd have to reschedule. Mum and I drove home in silence.

Amazingly, I just suddenly turned and spoke to her. Yes, my voice spontaneously came back! I just started carrying on a conversation with Mum. She didn't say, "Oh look you're talking," she knew the best thing was to just keep talking and not draw attention to it. Just calmly carry on a conversation. My voice was a bit weak but it was working!! After nine months of silence, I could finally speak!

I am convinced, with my positive thinking for the three weeks prior to my appointment, plus the visualisation in the hospital, I cured myself. I continued with voice coaching for three months to strengthen my unused throat muscles.

I know that focussing on your successful outcome, and all the things you could be doing with your outcome helps bring it about. Thinking positive thoughts really does promote good health and ultimate body function. I know. I did it for myself. Now I'm here to help you do the same. We'll work on making the most of what you've got: the whole package, the exercise, the eating and the mind. Anything is possible. I'm so passionate about helping you.

Part 1

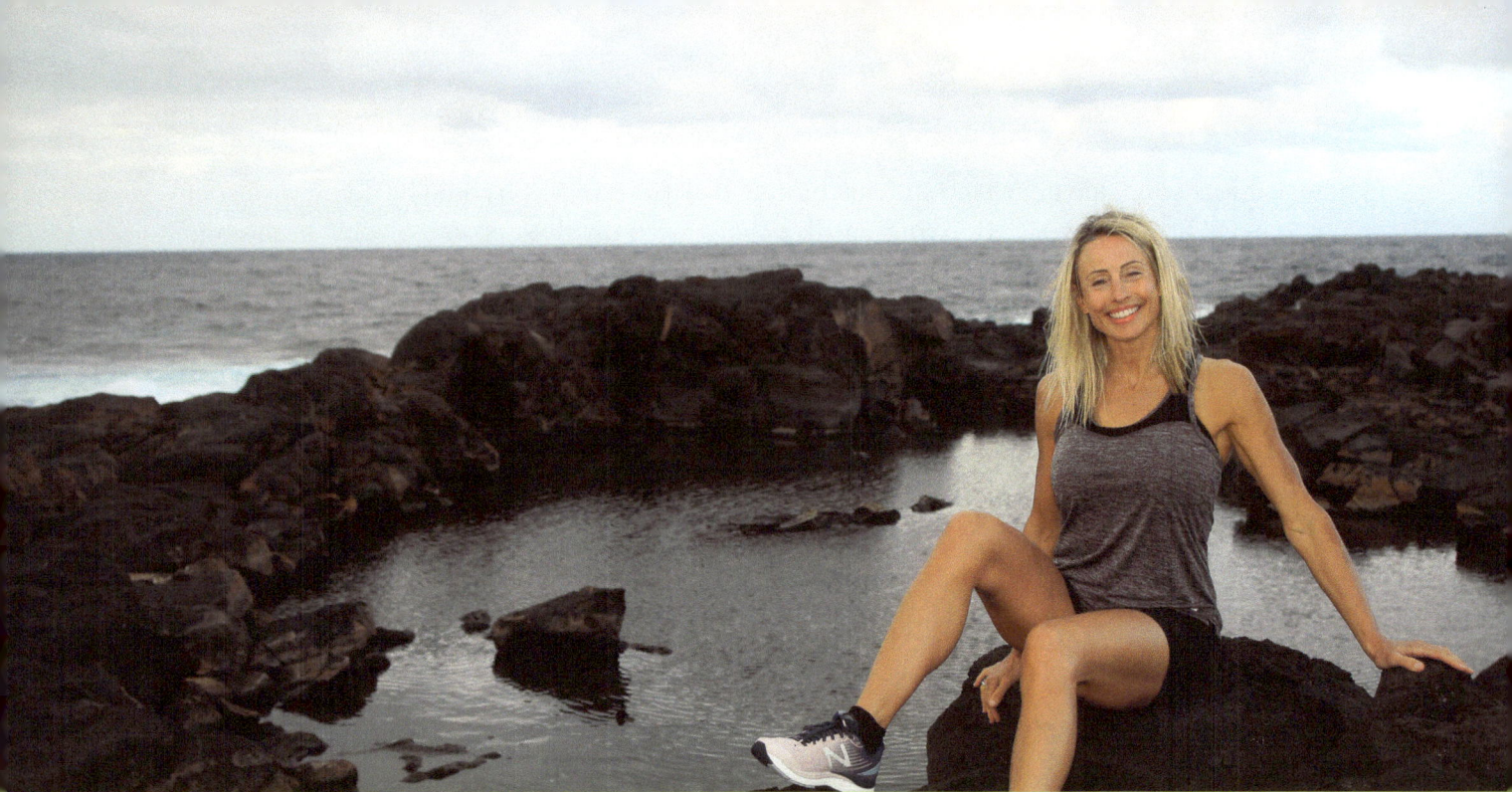

Your Pre-plan Work

Aperitif - Introduction

Your Best Body Ever is designed to deliver an exceptional, uncomplicated way of looking after yourself with a brilliant five point daily plan; helping you to live longer, fitter, happier and healthier. The plan looks at the whole solution incorporating physical and mental fitness, nutrition and steps toward a greater, happier and more enriched life. A refreshing change is yours for the taking, and remember, keep an open mind throughout.

So, what's happened? Have we forgotten how to look after ourselves? Have we been brain washed with mass advertising to live and eat in a certain way? Do we have to wait for a health problem to show up or a loved one to die before we wake up? Maybe, we've just got used to feeling tired all the time and consider that normal? Perhaps fed up with feeling old and everything is going south? Maybe your confidence isn't great, maybe it's even at its lowest level. You may have experienced signs of neglect showing up in your body which triggered the need to do something. Has there been a drama? Have you been dumped and just want to feel good about yourself? Or luckily, you may have landed a bit of free time to finally start to look after yourself properly. Are you frustrated there's never enough time to look after yourself?

Are you ready to take a stand and make a conscious decision to do something about the way you feel? Yes, I know, we're all time strapped, busy, pressured, have bills to pay, long hours at work and loads of things on the 'to do' list, But with a little persistent work on a daily basis your body, your spirit house, will undoubtedly perform, thrive and function so much better. You'll improve the quality of your life and of your loved ones and all the people around you. Now isn't that worth a bit of concerted effort?

Sit back and relax as you'll be shown what to do with this foundation in body and mind care: a five point daily plan helping you to keep on track and flourish for the long term.

Can you imagine an Olympic athlete training on their own, no coach, no team, no support, no expertise and no structured training programme? What are the chances of winning a medal? How well do you think that athlete is going to perform and get any kind of result? Pretty slim, right? This book is designed to increase your chances of winning in your life. Imagine what your life would look and feel like with Olympic level effort? A simple, straight talking five point daily plan helping you to stick to healthy body and mind choices for the long term. Simply amazing!

Think of someone you hold dear and love very much. Now switch that love and energy to yourself. Remember to keep an open mind. Have you ever noticed that you're quite prepared to buy an expensive present for someone else but couldn't justify spending that sort of money on yourself? You'd be quite happy to give lots of time, energy and love to other people with minimal if not any for yourself? What if you were to put some love into yourself and be the best version of you? Do you think the same people would benefit from a better you?

We humans are on this astonishing planet for such a short time. Why not capitalise and have the best ride of your life? Your best possible life experience by making the most of your greatest assets, your amazing body and mind! What an amazing piece of kit it is. Your phenomenal body! Your Best Friend! Your Energy House! Your centre of the universe!

Remember to stay open, enjoy the planning, enjoy the journey and enjoy being in the new zone as you work on the new you.

Getting Ready for Your Five Point Daily Plan

FOOD FOR THOUGHT

Have you ever known someone or thought to yourself, really that person didn't need to go like that, if only they'd looked after themselves, changed their lifestyle, took the advice to relax and eat properly etc. It's astonishing how long a lot of folks leave it until it's either too late or a nasty health problem shows up. Until then, they put their head in the sand. The great news, at any stage, unless you're dead, is that you can start to make positive changes. Now.

THREE CLIENTS, THEIR STORIES

Sue

Age: 50 something

Sue, a young grandma felt completely stuck in a rut, she was lacking in confidence and feeling very unfit. She wasn't happy with the middle age spread developing and her clothes feeling tight. Her waistline was thicker and the weight was piling on.

"It was looking like I was going to lose my job which was very unsettling and causing another black cloud over my life. I'd tried lots of diets and classes, some too complicated, others just not realistic which I wasn't getting on with or had the will to stick to and only covered part of the problem. I was a bit worried that life was going to slip by and feeling frustrated. I wanted out of this rut and was running out of ideas."

The organised structure and daily exercises are easy to follow and I feel able to work at my own pace. I've come to enjoy planning out quality time for myself to carry out daily disciplines, which have become ingrained in my daily routine. My diary reminders are like my own best friend. Since working through *Your Best Body Ever* plan and working with Anna, my fitness levels have improved and I feel so healthy, even better than I did in my 20s! I feel so much more confident and able to do more. It's given me a new lease on life. I've dropped a clothes size and my waist has shrunk. I like what I see in the mirror! I went on holiday and actually wore a bikini. Not feeling self-conscious was such a revelation. I now enjoy every day, approach my life differently and have more belief in myself to make positive changes.

Vanessa Jackson
Age: 42

As a single mum with two teenaged children and three jobs, I was just about holding it together. One of my jobs as a bookkeeper meant I spent a lot of time sitting at a desk. I suffered from neck and back pain. I was totally neglecting myself, putting on weight, not eating properly and felt stressed out. I was worried I'd need to go back on antidepressants and wanted a natural solution.

I was initially concerned that I just wouldn't have the time to dedicate to looking after myself. Six months later the whole family are eating well. It's no extra effort to eat properly and I'm now in the habit of making good food choices.

Anna's whole plan is simple, straightforward and effective. I now have so much more energy and enjoy life more. As I've started to feel better about myself and seeing the good in people, I met my amazing boyfriend. He's so good with the kids, kind, fun and such a great support. He's even created a large home grown vegetable plot in the garden. I am so grateful for my amazing boyfriend. I feel strong, resilient and better able to ask and accept help now too. Devoting a bit of time to myself has transformed my life. My back and neck are much improved with the posture correction exercises. It's all so simple, effective and easy to stick to. Life is great. I'm so happy now.

Gina Taylor
Age: 48

High blood pressure was a massive issue for me. It was really bothering me that my whole family has a history of heart disease. I was getting rather concerned a heart attack or a stroke was in the cards. My blood pressure medication was making me feel sick and the last test on my kidneys and liver function revealed dangerous levels.

I was really feeling the strain. I started searching for a solution for better health and quality of life. I had nothing to lose and decided to go for it.

It was such a relief to find something easy to follow and do. I felt a lot less stressed as doing something positive about it was a real help.

As I followed Anna's healthy eating, exercising and positive mind exercises, my blood pressure has reduced significantly. My medication is at its lowest level which is a lot kinder for my kidneys and liver. I don't feel sick anymore and I anticipate being completely off medication. It comes as such relief to my family that they've all decided to follow the plan and work alongside me and support me.

RAISE A TOAST – DECISION

Congratulations! You've made a decision to get yourself geared up and look after your amazing piece of kit. Your magnificent body and your magnificent mind! That is worth raising a toast for and making a commotion about! Making a decision is powerful! Have you ever noticed when you've made a decision in the past it was almost a relief? Have you ever noticed that as soon as you've made a decision all your energy goes in a focussed direction toward that decision? Bravo, you made the right choice and after all, you're worth it.

CHATTER – HABITUAL BEINGS

Our habits either serve or sabotage our efforts to get to where we want to get to. We are habitual creatures and live, stand by and could even die by our habits. Habits are sneaky and just hang around, we take the same actions and do the same things day after day. Think about your morning routine: Alarm, hot drink, shower, brush teeth, commute to work, check the email etc. Our actions and thoughts are the same day in and day out. We've only got one chance in this amazing thing called life. Habits can be changed. Do you want to know the wonderful news? Once good habits have been formed and established, they're hard to break.

SPICE UP YOUR LIFE – GET CLEAR ON YOUR GOAL

Where do we start? SETTING A GOAL

We are goal orientated beings. We need to have the end in mind. Why's that? Well, imagine getting into your car on your driveway. Imagine starting the car up without knowing where you're going.

Do you get off the driveway? Maybe you're shrugging your shoulders and saying to yourself, I don't know where to go.

So, imagine again, same scenario, getting into your car with an important engagement to get to. You know exactly where you're going. You put the address into your navigation and away you go. On the way you experience a road block, diverted traffic and various hold ups but you still reach your destination because during the journey you know exactly where you're headed. You make the necessary adjustments to get back on course along the way. Not setting a goal target is like a ship without a rudder, you'll be going round in circles.

The more precise and crystal clear you make your goal the more precise the results. Taking action in the direction of your well clarified goal equals speed and maximum productivity. If you say you can you can. If you say you can't then you can't. Whatever target you set your mind to, decide you can.

Here are some examples of extremely clear goals:

- Lose 6kg in 3 months
- Run a 10k in 53 minutes for my next event in 2 months time
- Come off anti-depressants in 6 months
- Get my body healthy so I can conceive this year
- Improve my skin
- Improve my energy levels
- Get off the sofa without using the armrests
- Get my pre-baby body back in 3 months
- Feel more confident

I've mentioned road blocks on your journey to your goal in the physical sense and your thinking can also slow you down or leave you sitting in your driveway. What's the best way of busting through our thinking, advancing off our driveway? For starters, be aware that such a thing exists.

So, we've made a decision, we've set a clear goal, we're aware we have some habits which either serve or sabotage our progress and we want to get to the next step.

On a scale of 1-5 How committed are you to succeed?

1 (not committed)   2   3   4   5 (very committed)

DREAM FOR A BIT

Now imagine the new you. What are you doing, what are you wearing? What setting are you in? Who's with you? What fun things are you doing? Can you see your face aching with a ton of smiles?

Imagine your eyes sparkling, walking confidently with a spring in your step. Moving, looking and feeling amazing. Relishing every moment and enjoying being the better version of you.

Put an inspiring picture of you on the fridge, somewhere where you'll see it every day. A previous picture of you or an inspirational photo of someone you admire. Someone you aspire to look like, be like. Write out a written statement and put on the wall incorporating your goal target.

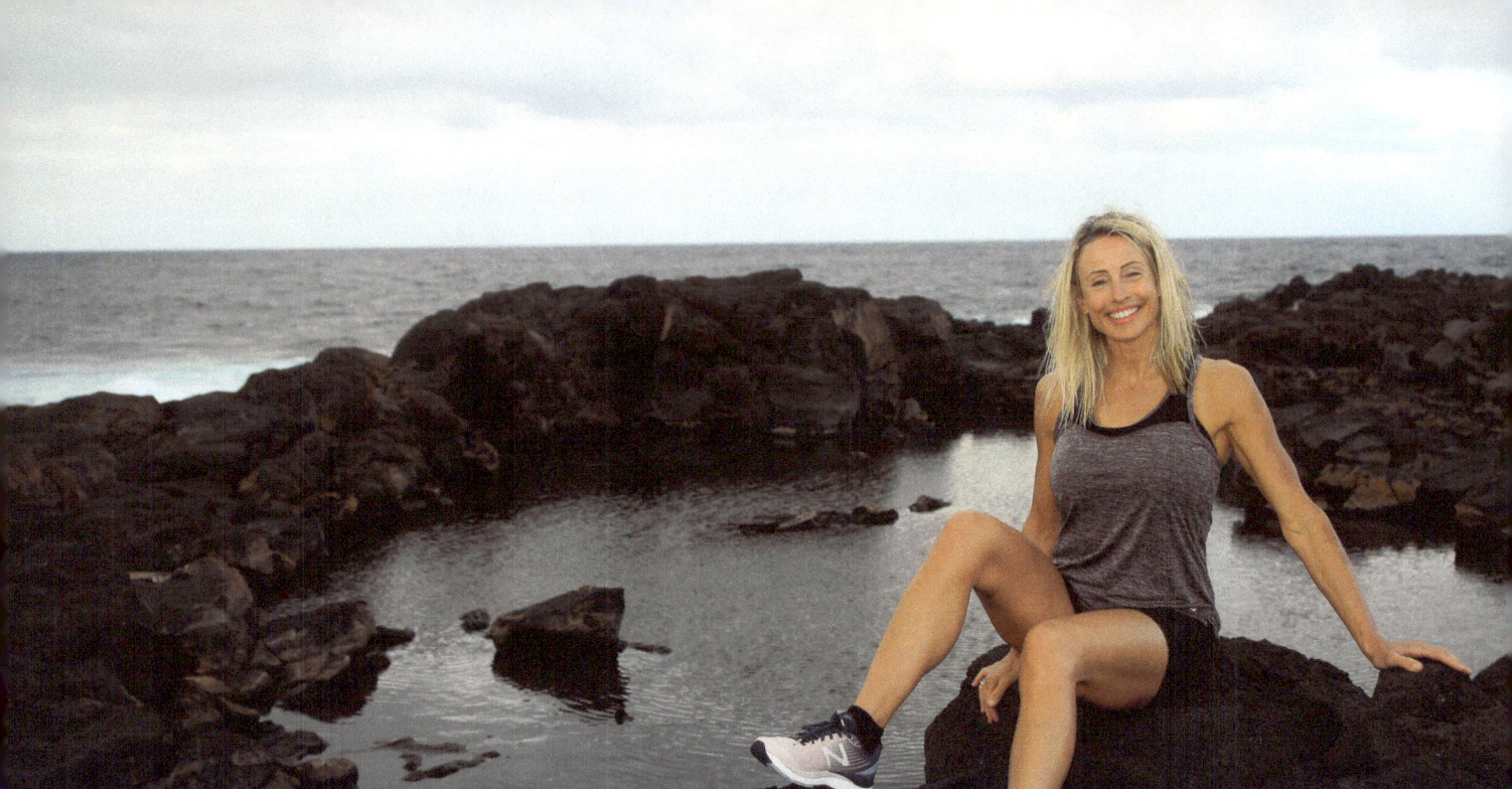

Part II

The Plan

Easy as 1, 2, 3, 4, 5

Unlock the hidden gems as you turn the pages describing the Five Point Daily Plan of your nourishing body and mind solution.

YOUR FIVE POINT DAILY PLAN

1. Cheers – Gratitude
2. Nature for Well-being
3. Best body fuel – balanced meals
4. Nourishing Mind Questions - Happiness boosters
5. Best Body 5 Components of Fitness Routines

STEP 1. Cheers – Gratitude

Raise your glass, a toast, appreciating all things to be grateful for. A toast to celebrate all the good in your life and all the good on its way to you.

As you start to think of the wonderful experiences, people and blessings to be grateful for you'll attract more of the same. Gratitude creates harmony with the sweet level of life and forms an attractive force, magnetising love, happiness and bliss your way. It brings you more of the good stuff.

Impress gratitude on your mind, appreciate and be so eternally grateful for all the good in your life. You get to live another magnificent day, the best day of your life, be grateful for your loved ones, your great health, fitness and be so grateful for the sheer beauty of each moment.

To help you to the sweet place of feeling grateful write a list of 5 things you're grateful for first thing in the morning. See the reference section at the back for some examples. Make up your own or copy from some examples that resonate with you. Allow yourself some quiet time with your thoughts and allow wonderful grateful feelings to expand to over flowing within you.

STEP 2. Nature for well-being – marvel at beauty whilst walking

Every day aim to walk in nature or a park as vibrations from plants and trees work in harmony with us to create a lovely, well-being vibe in the body. Aim for half an hour, but if you can only manage 15 minutes, even such a short burst will add a real boost to calm and happiness.

Exercising outside with nature close helps to clear out the lungs and is the ultimate for body exhilaration, alertness and freshness. Walking is good for digestion and bowel movement in the removing of toxins from the body. When out walking in nature notice your breathing and how lovely it is to recognise just how amazing your body is and what a wondrous world we live in.

Another great tip is to have lots of beautiful houseplants to continue nature's magic in your home. We feel more at home in nature, our more natural environment. Plants, trees and places of outstanding natural beauty are good for us. Allow yourself some nature time. Plants, trees and nature soften out any tension too. Some businesses have cottoned onto this concept and decked out their offices with fake grass, sheep and beautiful nature landscapes in pictures and painted walls. Apparently, productivity and wellness in the office increases by as much as 20% with nature being added to the office interior.

STEP 3. Best body – Balanced Meals

Make 5 best decisions around balanced eating, drinking 2.5 litres of water and keeping to portion size each day and for each meal.

5 Best Decision Points

1. Best Carbs
2. Best Proteins
3. Best fats
4. 2.5 litres water
5. Portion size

This is not about denial, but eating nutrient rich foods that will keep you feeling full longer. This is not meant as a quick fix diet but a lifestyle and good choice maker. You shouldn't feel starving and lacking in anything. Nutrient rich foods give your body what it needs to feel satisfied and replenished. If you feed your body substandard food, the body's survival hunger hormone will more than likely be switched on, sending a message to the brain more food is needed in order to obtain the nutrients it really requires. Your body is not satisfied when it is presented with nutrient deficient food. Substandard food (lacking in nutrients), more often than not results in overeating.

Your best body fuel is comprised of three balanced meals per day. Include best carbs, best protein and best fats. A meal is defined as food going into your mouth and includes snacks. The ideal is to eat three balanced meals per day without snacking. However, if you have to snack there are healthy snack options suggested in the reference section.

A gap between meals aids digestion. The body uses a lot of energy to digest food, so a gap between meals improves energy levels too. To get the balance right using the right combination of nutrients aim for each meal portion size and components to be measured as follows: good carbs (double cupped hands, piled up), good protein (size and depth of the palm of your hand), good fats (half to full thumb size).

You don't need to weigh food, look at calories or use reduced fat products. You just need to make the right choices. Go for natural, whole, organic, non-processed foods. When eating your nutritious, naturally balanced meal, aim to chew your food 30-50 times per mouthful. Chewing your food not only aids digestion, but you'll feel full sooner and be encouraged to eat less.

Remember to always drink plenty of water every day (at least 2.5 litres) as water improves mood, energy levels and you'll be more alert as a consequence. Your brain is 80% water. Your body averages 70%, so water is absolutely essential for ultimate body function, health and vitality. Be sure to drink water 15-30 minutes before eating a meal as an aid to filling you up and encouraging you to eat less.

BEST CARBS (Carbohydrates)

Best Non-starchy Vegetables: broccoli, carrots, cauliflower, spinach, mushrooms, celery, peppers (green, red & yellow), onions, lettuce, water cress, cucumber, asparagus, garlic and herbs.

Best Starchy vegetables: pumpkin/squash, swede, turnips, beetroot, sweet potato, corn on the cob, leeks and new boiled potatoes with skins on.

Best Fruit: lemon, lime, avocado, tomato, grapefruit, blueberries and apples

Best grains: brown rice, quinoa and buckwheat

Try to eat fewer grains and fruits and more vegetables for your carb portion.

A colourful food plate gives you a greater range and concentration of phytochemicals for good health.

BEST PROTEINS

Best plant based protein: quinoa, soya, chia seeds, tofu, chickpeas and raw nuts and seeds.

Best Fish: salmon, tuna, swordfish, trout and halibut

Best dairy: organic free range eggs

Best meat: organic chicken, organic turkey, organic pork, organic beef and wild duck

Use less meat in your diet. Completely avoid all processed meat such as ham, bacon, sausages and salami.

BEST FATS

Best fats: organic coconut oil, organic extra virgin olive oil, organic unsalted butter and naturally occurring fat in raw nuts (such as almonds, walnuts and brazil nuts), raw seeds, avocado and fresh olives

There's a best food shopping list and recipes in line with best balanced meals both with and without meat (vegetarian and vegan) in the reference section at the end of this book.

STEP FOUR. Nourishing Mind Questions – Happiness booster

As human beings we have the ability to think. We can choose to have happy thoughts, positive thoughts, fun and playful thoughts. With practice we have the ability to immediately switch from non-positive thoughts to positive thoughts. Positive, enriching thoughts directed in this way help improve the quality of your life. By directing your thoughts, actions and feelings in a positive way you are setting up a mirror, an attractive force to reflect the positive to come right back at you. It may not happen immediately and quite often comes back from different people or situations at a different time. On the flip side, you'll tend to find negative thoughts, actions and feelings come back almost immediately. Plus, it's really hard work and tiring to think negatively and in no way serves you at all. To help bring your thinking right back on track and steer your thoughts in a happy, positive, purposeful, harmonious, heart-felt and loving way ask these five questions of yourself every day:

1. What can I do today to be the best version of me?
2. What's going to serve me best with this meal choice?
3. What praise worthy feedback can I give myself?
4. What praise can I give this person in front of me?
5. What could be added to make this moment even more perfect?

Have these questions at the forefront of your mind as you go about your day. They can be used at any time, fitting into your day and your thoughts to help make the most of yourself, benefit you and benefit the people around you. Every day be aware of the questions and use them when appropriate. They are a running theme when you have moments to yourself in your own thoughts or have someone in front of you.

Here's an example to help you see how you can put these magical questions into your day.

You've just started stirring and waking up and think to yourself *how grateful I am that I get to live another wonderful day.*

You're brushing your teeth, looking in the mirror and asking yourself **What can I do today to be the best version of me?** (You could even write a note *What can I do today to be the best version of me?* and stick it on the wall/mirror in your bathroom as a prompt).

www.annascanlan.com

Whilst brushing your teeth, you think about the person you want to be to help get you get one step closer to your goal and be the best version of you. You think, *Okay, so today I am going to smile a lot, have a positive attitude, see the good in people, look after my amazing body* and have a positive impact on everybody I meet.

You're looking around the supermarket planning your next couple of future healthy meals and constantly thinking **What's going to serve me with this meal choice?**

You head toward the organic fruit and vegetable section and pick up a colourful array of salad and vegetables to go with your next few meals. You're in line at the till and decide you're going to find a way to praise the teller. **What praise can I give this person in front of me?** The cashier gives a big warm smile, has a friendly and helpful disposition and provides a smooth, efficient service and you're so impressed the praise comes easily and you go overboard with praise directed at the friendly cashier and thank them very much.

As you're driving back from the supermarket and getting to the last few blocks toward home, a magnificent red sky presents itself. You can't help but to notice just how beautiful it is. **What could be added to make this moment even more perfect?** You get to tap into your imagination, have fun transporting yourself to dream land. For example, you could see yourself walking hand in hand with your soul mate on a beautiful, lush mountain path with exotic birds singing. You feel peaceful and loving and smiling up into this magnificent red sky. You turn to your soul mate, locking in with a long lingering heart felt look into each other eyes.

You're just about to pull into your driveway when you spot your neighbour out front tending to a flowerbed in their garden. **What praise can I give this person in front of me?**

You complement your neighbour's pretty garden and how neat and beautifully tended it is. (Goes without saying, only praise when you mean it. People can tell if praise isn't genuine).

The family meal you prepare that evening made up of fresh ingredients, lots of tasty herbs and goodness is a real hit with the family. You've also completed all the 5 steps of *Your Best Body Ever*. **What praiseworthy feedback can I give myself?** Well done (your name) what a phenomenal cook you are! Fist pump! So creative and talented in the kitchen. Woo hoo I'm living my best life ever and am proud of my magnificent body and mind and how well I take care of it.

This is pure fantasy; however, I hope you get the idea. It's your day, your life, enjoy, chuckle and have fun as you go along. Live and be experiencing your best Life with your 5 questions.

STEP 5. Fitness Best Body 5 Components of Fitness Routines

Complete just one five minute workout from your Best Body 5 different workout routines

You'll find five varied workouts, each touching the components of fitness. The idea here is to help your body move, look and feel better. These five workouts, each five minutes long with five exercise blocks a piece, include the exercises below:

Scan QR Code to visit **yourbestbodyever.com** and view the video workouts.

1) Posture alignment (5 minutes)

- Release the back of your neck – push your chin into your neck with your first two fingers (60 seconds)

- Tilt head to side, gently assist with hand (30 seconds each side)

- Pec/Chest opener using a doorway (both arms 60 seconds) or post (each arm 30 seconds each side)

- Soft knee wall sit – Flatten lower back to wall, chin in, shoulders back, back of head on wall and hold (60 seconds)

- Back activator – Lie on floor, arms straight in front by ears, look at floor, switch on bum muscles throughout, lead with thumbs as you take arms back. Back and forth with arms. (60 seconds)

2) Stretching/Relax (5 minutes)

- Alternate arm stretch –stretch to the sky, standing (60 seconds)

- Pigeon – make an arrow with your right knee, hands either side of knee, other leg is straight going back, gently lean forward. Swap sides. Make an arrow with your left knee, hands either side of knee, gently lean forward, other leg straight back (30 seconds each side)

- Downward Dog (60 seconds)

- Cobra into Swan (2 x 30 seconds)
- Lunge with side stretch – left leg forward with right arm stretching over sideways, switch legs, right leg forward with left arm over sides ways (30 seconds each side)

3) Core/Midsection (5 minutes)

- Plank on elbows (60 seconds)
- Dead bug – lie on back, stack knees over hips and arms over shoulders, take opposite arm back and leg forward, alternate leg and arm within a few inches of touching the floor (60 seconds)
- Side plank on elbow (30 seconds each side)
- Kick ups (60 seconds)
- Lie down mini crunch (60 seconds)

4) Controlled body weight exercises (5 minutes)

- Snake press up (60 seconds)
- Squat with feet shoulder width apart (60 seconds)
- Table top with butt improver – sit tall, knees bent, hands by sides, fingers facing forward. In control continuously bring hips up to table top, squeeze butt at top then back down (60 seconds)
- Alternate lunge into knee hug (60 seconds)
- Bear crawl as low as you can go – back and forth (60 seconds)

5) High Energy Burst (5 minutes)

- Running arms (30 seconds, change leading foot)
- Split jump (60 seconds)
- Mountain climbers (60 seconds)
- Square jump (30 seconds each direction)
- Touch floor jumping stars (60 seconds)

Keep working through the workouts in the following order.

Monday – Posture alignment (5 minutes)

Tuesday – Stretching/relax (5 minutes)

Wednesday – Core/Midsection (5 minutes)

Thursday – Controlled body weight exercises (5 minutes)

Friday – High Energy Burst (5 minutes)

Saturday – Posture alignment (5 minutes)

Sunday – Stretching/relax (5 minutes)

1 Posture alignment (5 minutes)

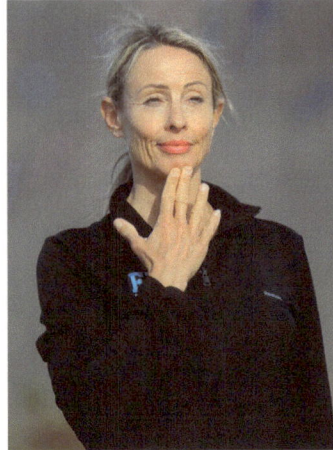

Release the back of your neck – push your chin into your neck with your first two fingers (60 seconds)

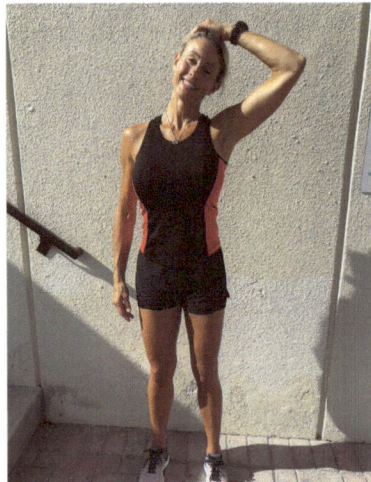

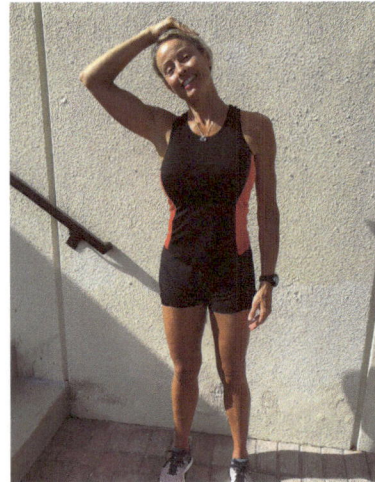

Tilt head side to side – gently assist with hand (30 seconds each side)

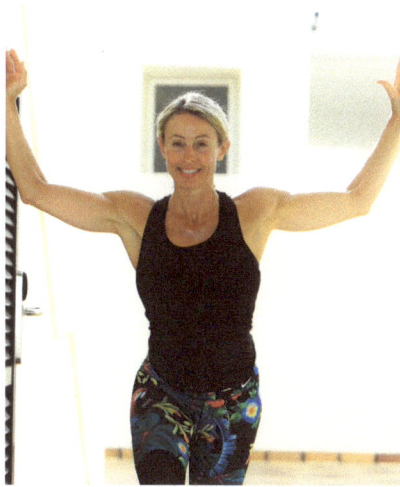

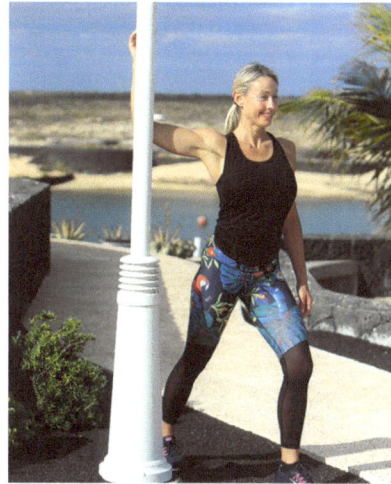

Pec/Chest opener – using a doorway (both arms 60 seconds) or post (each arm 30 seconds each side)

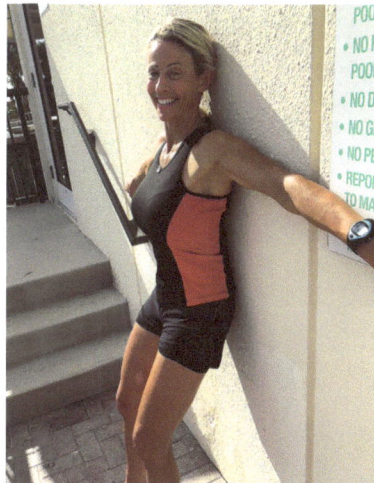

Soft knee wall sit – Flatten lower back to wall, chin in, shoulders back, back of head on wall and hold (60 seconds)

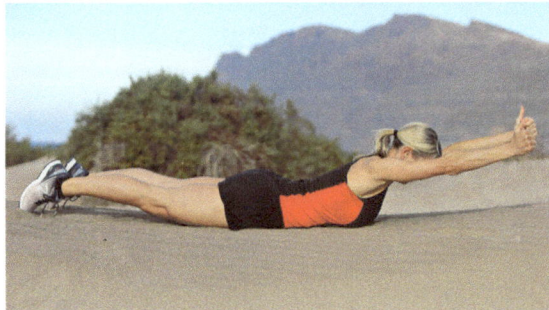

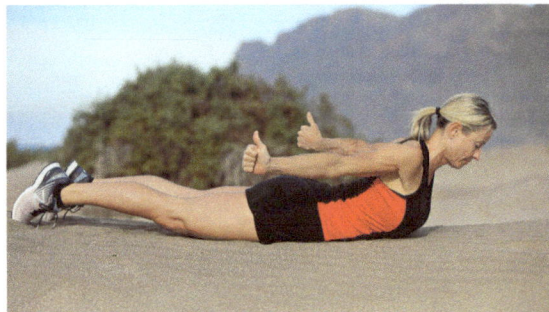

Back activator – Lie on floor, arms straight in front by ears, look at floor, switch on bum muscles throughout, lead with thumbs as you take arms back. Back and forth with arms. (60 seconds)

2 Stretching/Relax (5 minutes)

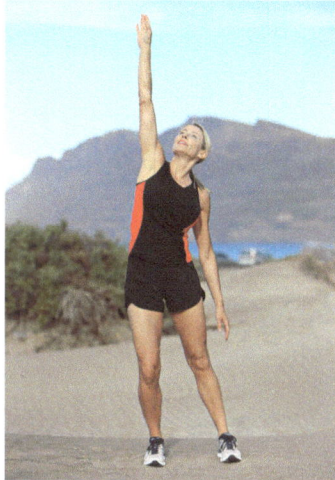

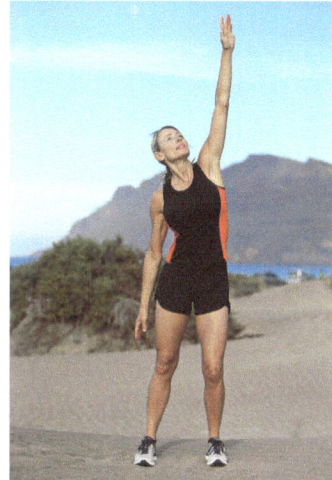

Alternate arm stretch – stretch to the sky, standing (60 seconds)

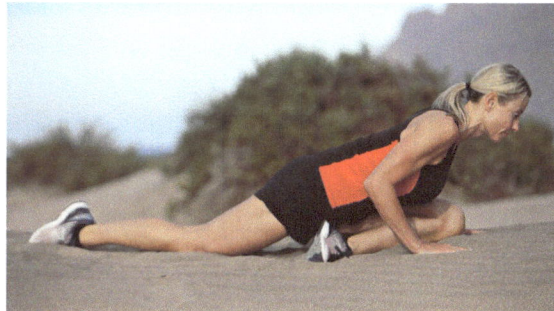

Pigeon – make an arrow with your right knee, hands either side of knee, other leg is straight going back, gently lean forward. Swap sides. Make an arrow with your left knee, hands either side of knee, gently lean forward, other leg straight back (30 seconds each side)

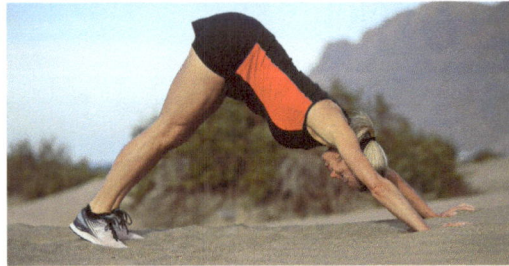

Downward Dog – (60 seconds)

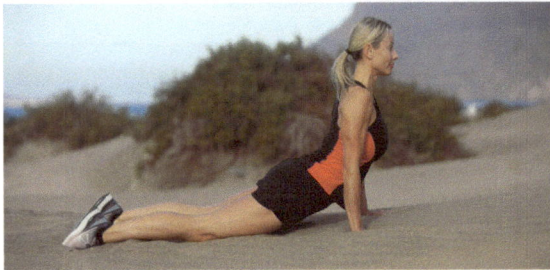

Cobra (30 seconds)

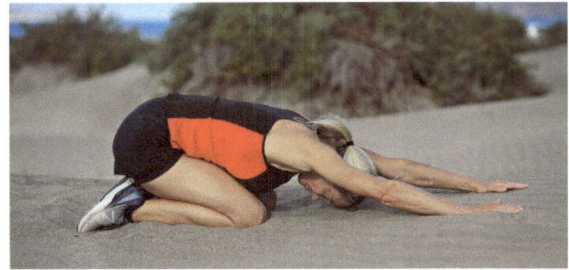

Into swan – (30 seconds)

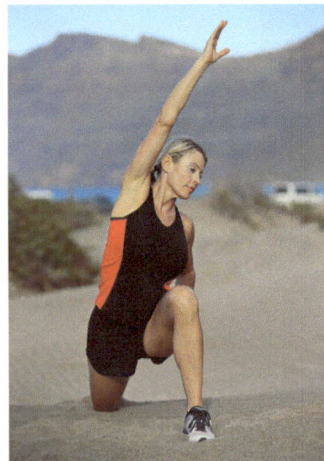

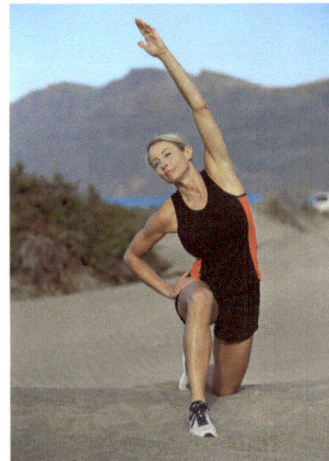

Lunge with side stretch – left leg forward with right arm stretching over sideways, switch legs, right leg forward with left arm over sides ways (30 seconds each side)

3 Core/Midsection (5 minutes)

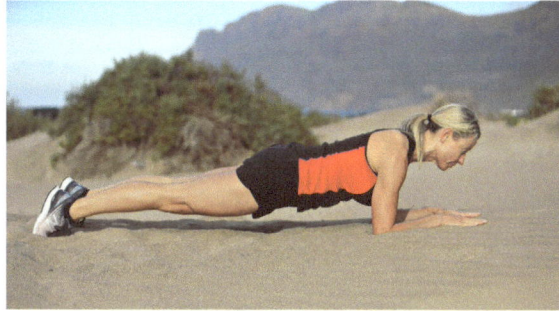

Plank on elbows – (60 seconds)

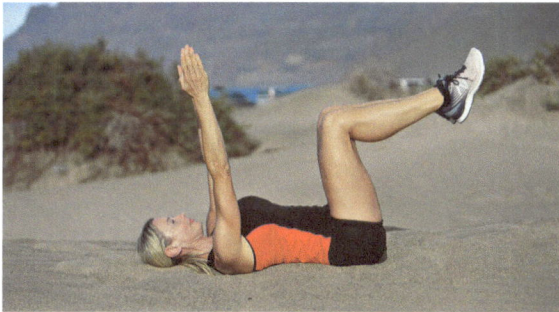

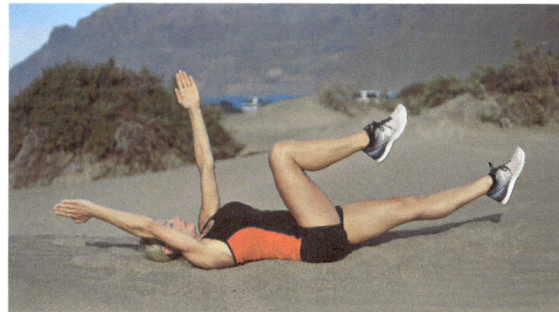

Dead bug – lie on back, stack knees over hips and arms over shoulders, take opposite arm back and leg forward, alternate leg and arm within a few inches of touching the floor (60 seconds)

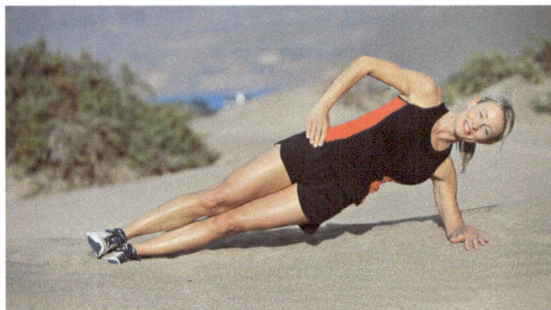

Side plank on elbow – (30 seconds each side)

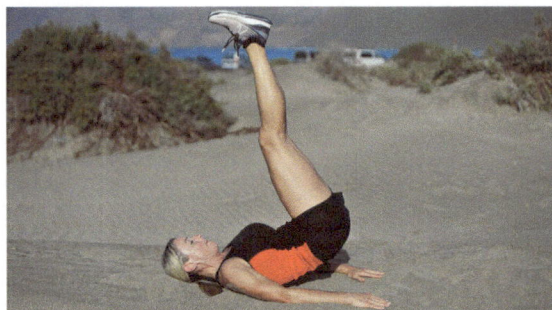

Kick ups – (60 seconds)

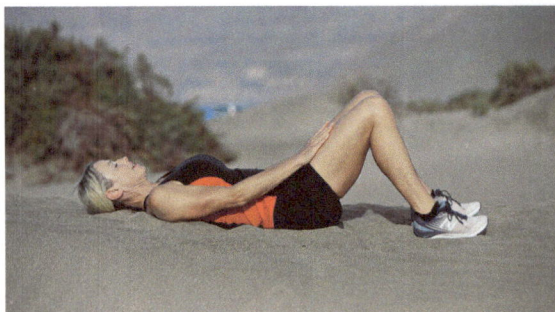

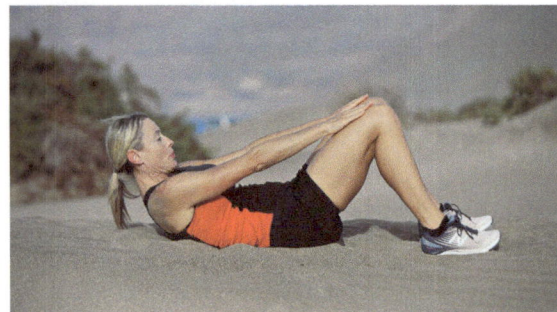

Lie down mini crunch – (60 seconds)

4 Controlled body weight exercises (5 minutes)

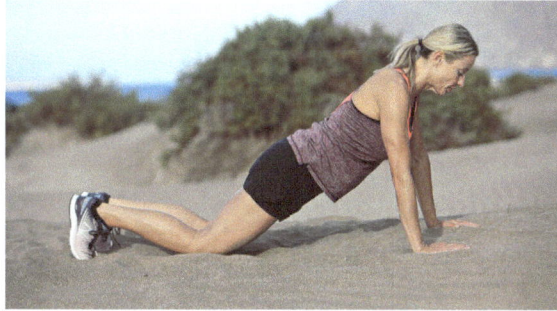

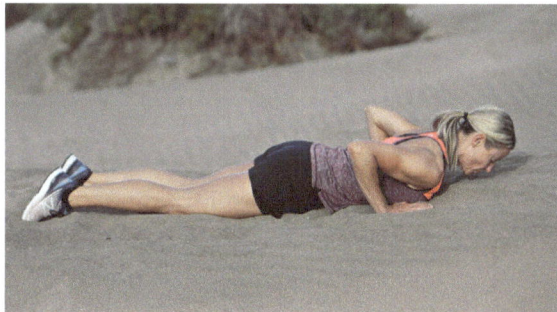

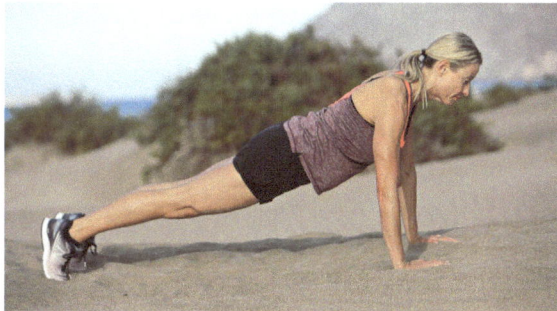

Snake press up – (60 seconds)

www.annascanlan.com

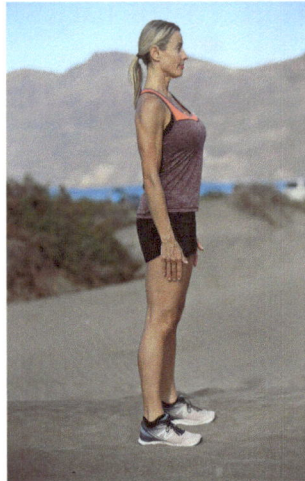

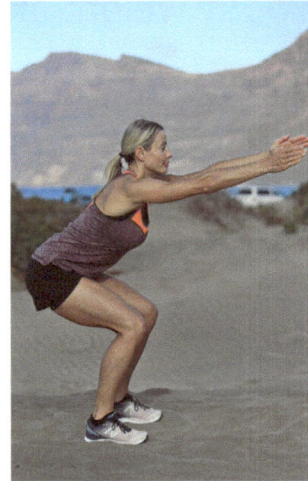

Squat – with feet shoulder width apart (60 seconds

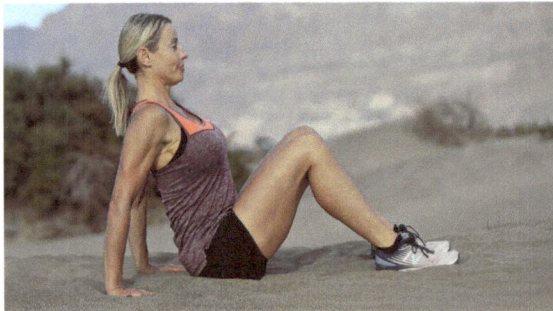

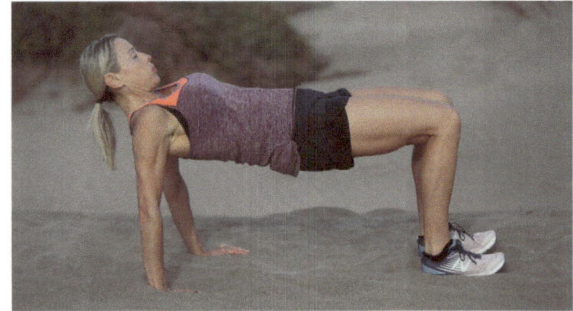

Table top with butt improver – sit tall, knees bent, hands by sides, fingers facing forward. In control continuously bring hips up to table top, squeeze butt at top then back down (60 seconds)

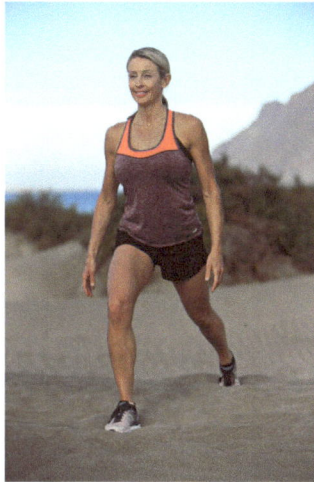

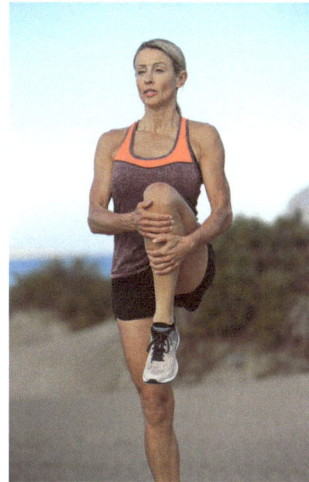

Alternate lunge – into knee hug (60 seconds)

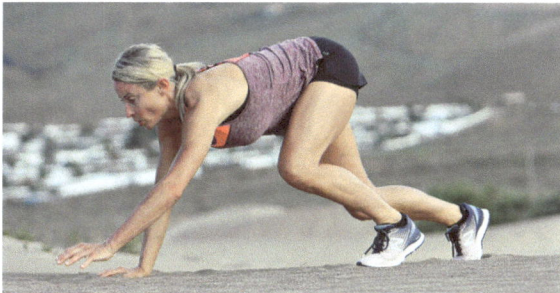

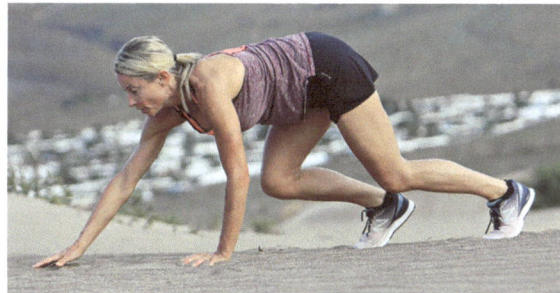

Bear crawl – as low as you can go – back and forth (60 seconds)

5 High Energy Burst (5 minutes)

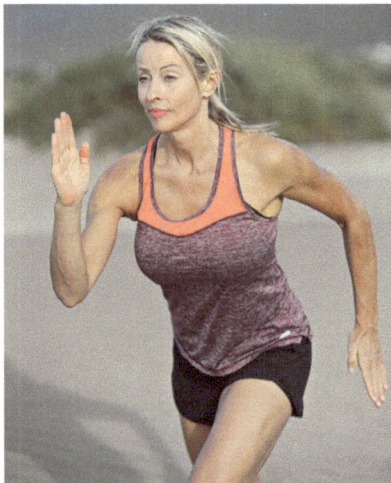

Running arms – (30 seconds, change leading foot)

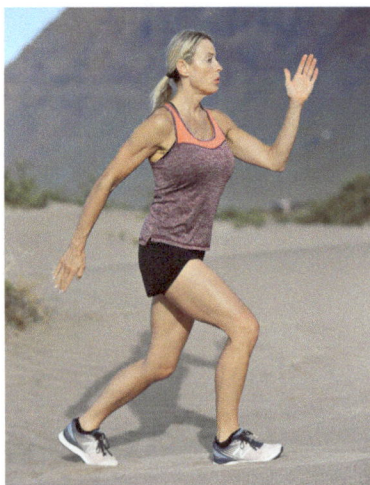

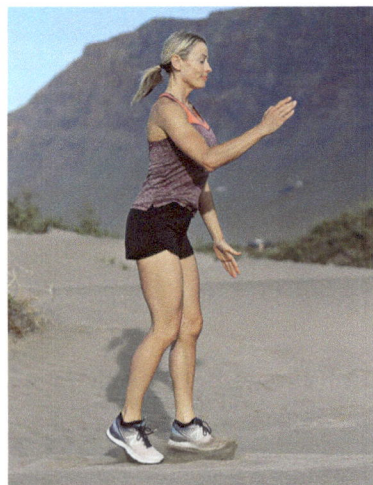

Split jump – (60 seconds)

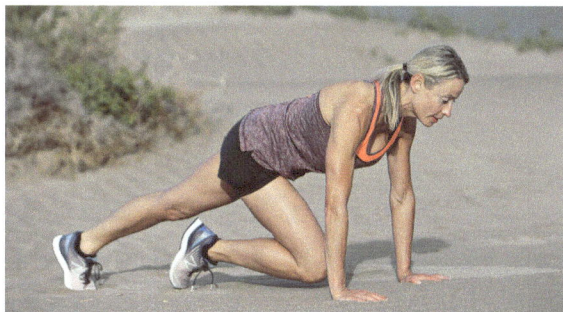

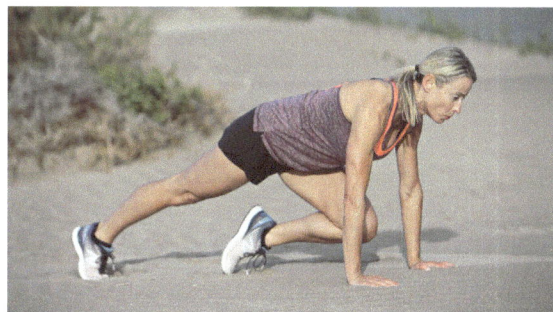

Mountain climbers – (60 seconds)

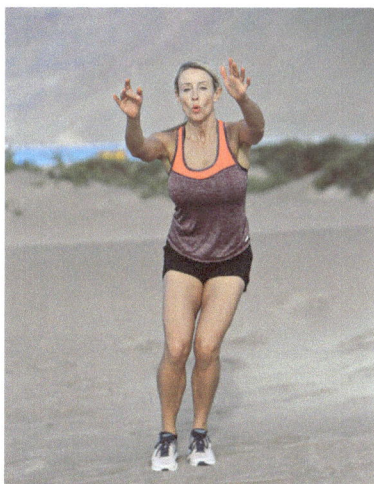

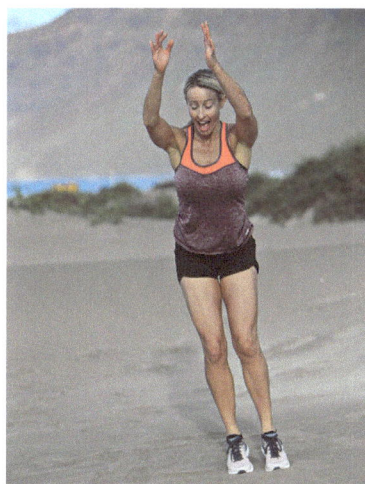

Square jump – (30 seconds each direction)

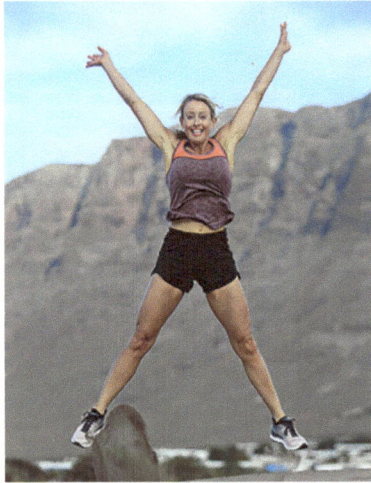

Touch floor jumping stars – (60 seconds)

HABIT RE-PROGRAMMING

Now that you've decided on your goal, you're committed to forming some new daily habits to reach that goal. These habits help you create and make the most of life in a fit, happy, healthy body.

You're now familiar with the five key points you'll be working on every day. This is your chance to engage and take action in daily disciplines specially designed to help make the most of life. This work will result in good choices being second nature to you and giving you the edge to win every day.

MAKING THE MOST OF YOUR DAILY FIVE POINT PLAN

Your set yourself up for success check list:

1. Here's a one-time task before you start, plug daily prompts into your electronic diary with a 30 minute reminder. Set prompts on repeat for every day.

Here's an example of what your daily prompts look like:

7am – Five things you're grateful for.

8am – Best Mind question – *What can I do today to be the best version of me?*

9am – Best Mind question – *What's going to serve me best with this meal choice?*

10am – Best Mind question – *What praise worthy feedback can I give myself?*

Noon – Best Mind question – *What's going to serve me best with this meal choice?*

1pm – Walk in Nature/Appreciate Nature

2pm – Best Mind question – *What praise can I give this person in front of me?*

3pm – Best Mind question – *What could be added to make this moment even more perfect?*

5pm – Best Mind question – *What's going to serve me best with this meal choice?*

6pm – Best body 5 Fitness

7pm – *What praise worthy feedback can I give myself?*

8pm – Mark my progress – grades for the day

2. At the end of each day, grade yourself on how you feel and your level of effort and application on each of the 5 points using the scale below.

0 Disappointing

1 Poor

2 Reasonable effort

3 Above average

4 Superb work

5 Outstanding/Winner!

Scan this QR code to visit **yourbestbodyever.com** to access and download your grading table document.

There's an opportunity to increase your Best Body 5 Components of Fitness Routines by adding three routines together (1 Star) or all five routines together (2 stars).

Best combinations to earn 1 star:

Posture alignment + Stretching/Relax + Core

Posture alignment + Stretching/Relax + Controlled Body Weight

Posture alignment + Stretching/relax + High Energy Burst

Best combination to earn 2 Stars:

Run through all five components of fitness routines

Posture alignment + Stretching/Relax + Core + Controlled Body Weight + High Energy Burst

Monday	Tuesday	Wednesday	Thursday	Friday	Saturday	Sunday
Gratitude List 5	Gratitude List 5	Gratitude List 5	Gratitude List 5	Gratitude List 5	Gratitude List 5	Gratitude List 5
Walk in nature	Walk in nature	Walk in nature	Walk in nature	Walk in nature	Walk in nature	Walk in nature
Best Body Fuel Balance 2.5 litre water Portion size	Best Body Fuel Balance 2.5 litre water Portion size	Best Body Fuel Balance 2.5 litre water Portion size	Best Body Fuel Balance 2.5 litre water Portion size	Best Body Fuel Balance 2.5 litre water Portion size	Best Body Fuel Balance 2.5 litre water Portion size	Best Body Fuel Balance 2.5 litre water Portion size
Nourishing Mind Questions – Happiness Boosters x 5	Nourishing Mind Questions – Happiness Boosters x 5	Nourishing Mind Questions – Happiness Boosters x 5	Nourishing Mind Questions – Happiness Boosters x 5	Nourishing Mind Questions – Happiness Boosters x 5	Nourishing Mind Questions – Happiness Boosters x 5	Nourishing Mind Questions – Happiness Boosters x 5
Best Body 5 Components of Fitness Routines 5 mins ☐ +1 star ☐ +2 stars	Best Body 5 Components of Fitness Routines 5 mins ☐ +1 star ☐ +2 stars	Best Body 5 Components of Fitness Routines 5 mins ☐ +1 star ☐ +2 stars	Best Body 5 Components of Fitness Routines 5 mins ☐ +1 star ☐ +2 stars	Best Body 5 Components of Fitness Routines 5 mins ☐ +1 star ☐ +2 stars	Best Body 5 Components of Fitness Routines 5 mins ☐ +1 star ☐ +2 stars	Best Body 5 Components of Fitness Routines 5 mins ☐ +1 star ☐ +2 stars

3. Complete the 5 points every day

Being graded has been instilled from our school days and appraisals are used in the work place. Grades serve as a great marker and checking system of progress. They're really motivating and help keep you on track. Staying focussed and determined with daily repetition is the best way to change your habits. It takes two to four months of consistent daily repetition to start making new habits second nature and the new normal. Keep with it.

As mentioned, when you end your day, finish up with grading yourself out of 5 for each of the 5 points of your daily plan. How about a little celebration for what you've achieved with a private fist punch or how about sharing with loved ones or good friends. Well done for your efforts. Praise yourself.

I always suggest gratitude first thing in the morning because getting on the right vibe of gratitude is a phenomenal start to your day. The remaining points: walk in Nature, Best Body Fuel, Best Mind Questions and Best Body 5 min workout are time flexible, you can work them in to suit you at any time of day.

FINAL THOUGHTS

Remember when you learned to drive? You were consciously aware of every move you made. You had to really think and concentrate on what you were doing: changing gears, checking the mirror, pressing the accelerator, using the brake, checking road signs and indicating. There was a lot to take in and get in smooth sequence and combination. When you passed your test, gained some experience and knew what you were doing, your driving became more natural and automatic. You didn't even have to think about it. The same principle applies to your daily plan. Keep going with your daily points, every day. Once you get through the clunky stage of consciously having to think about what you're doing, it's likely you'll transition into your new, normal healthy habits.

ANOTHER FINAL THOUGHT

Imagine you wanted to develop a muscular physique. You went to the gym, did an all nighter and worked out all through the weekend. You expected to get a muscular physique by putting in such a concentrated effort. What are the chances of that working? Pretty slim right? Not going to happen.

On the reverse approach, to get long term, lasting results for your physical body, your mental muscle and your habits you must continue on a daily basis all the points of your 5 point plan. I strongly recommend you stay laser focussed and keep it going for a minimum of two months to make that shift.

Good luck, you're on the right path. Let me know how you're getting on.

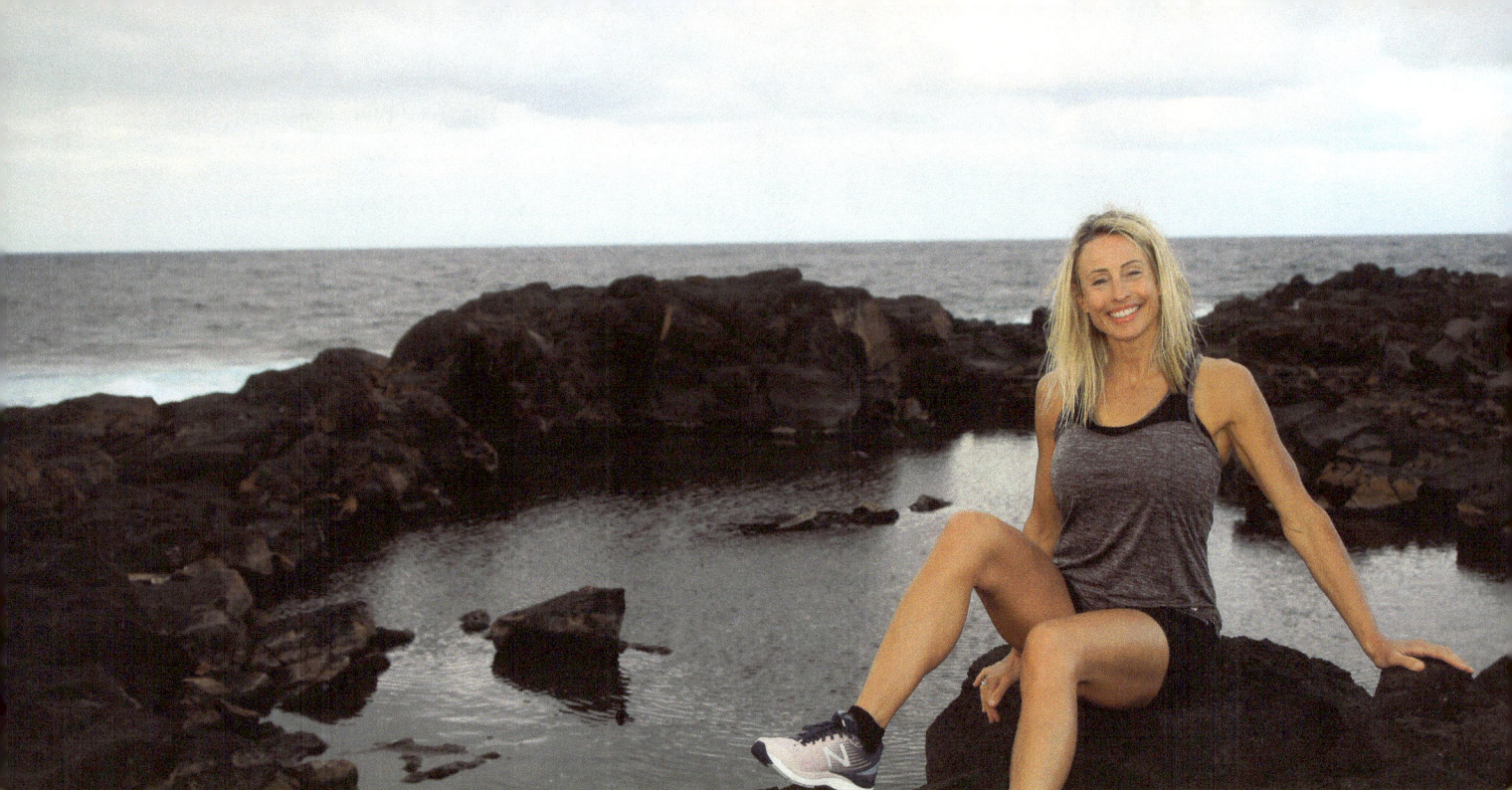

Part III

Recipes

RECIPES

LEEK AND SWEET POTATO SOUP (VEGETARIAN & VEGAN)

Serves 4

1 Medium onion, finely chopped

1 tablespoon coconut oil

1 leek, finely sliced

1 medium sweet potato diced. Scrub and leave skin on.

1 teaspoon ground cumin

1.5 litres (2 pints) organic vegetable stock

100g (3 ½ oz) quinoa

1 clove garlic, peeled and left whole

Instructions

Soften the onion in a tablespoon of coconut oil in a large saucepan.

Add the leek and sweet potato and cook for 2 minutes.

Add the cumin, pour in the stock and simmer for 15 minutes.

Simmer two parts water to one part quinoa in a separate saucepan for 15 minutes.

Pour in quinoa and any remaining stock, liquidise with a hand blender and serve.

MILD CURRIED CHICKPEA & VEGETABLE SOUP (VEGETARIAN & VEGAN)

Serves 2

1 tablespoon coconut oil

1 large onion, finely chopped

½ teaspoon mild curry powder

1 tablespoon tomato puree

1 head broccoli (250g / 9oz approximately) cut into small florets

2 sticks celery, chopped

2 carrots, scrub, leave skins on and chop into small pieces

1 litre (2 pints) vegetable stock

1 200g (7oz) can chickpeas

Instructions

Heat the oil in a large saucepan and sauté the onion with the curry power for 3-4 minutes.

Add the tomato puree, broccoli, celery and carrot and stir continuously over a high heat for 4 minutes.

Add the vegetable stock, bring to a boil and simmer for 15 minutes.

Rinse and drain the chickpeas and add them to the soup.

Cook for a further 5 minutes.

Allow to cool sufficiently so you can liquidize with a hand blender.

Heat through and serve with soda bread, rye bread, pumpernickel bread, oatcakes or wheat free/gluten free/yeast free bread.

SPICED CARROT & LENTIL SOUP (VEGETARIAN & VEGAN)

Serves 2

2 teaspoons cumin seeds

½ teaspoon chili flakes

2 teaspoons organic coconut oil

600g carrots, coarsely grated

150g red lentils

725ml water

400ml can coconut milk

Himalayan Salt & pepper to taste

Coconut yogurt

Fresh Coriander

Instructions

Heat a large pan and dry fry the cumin seeds & chili flakes for 1 minute.

Put half of this mixture aside for later.

Add the coconut oil, carrot, lentils, water and coconut milk to the pan and bring to a boil.

Simmer for 20 minutes until the lentils have softened.

Pulse until smooth using a hand blender or liquidizer.

Season to taste with Himalayan salt and fresh ground black pepper.

Dress with coconut yogurt, sprinkle on the reserved roasted spices.

Add fresh coriander and serve.

TOMATO & ROSEMARY SOUP (VEGETARIAN & VEGAN)

Serves 2

1 medium onion, diced

2 stalks celery, sliced

1 carrot, diced

1 large clove garlic, crushed

1 400g (14oz) tinned chopped plum tomatoes

1 sprig fresh rosemary

Juice of one lemon

1 litre (1¾ pints) of vegetable stock

50g (2oz) shredded spinach

Instructions

Heat two tablespoons of olive oil in a large saucepan.

Add the onion, celery, carrot and garlic and cook gently over a low heat until the vegetables begin to soften.

Stir in the tomatoes and add the rosemary and lemon juice, stir in for a few minutes.

Add the stock and simmer for 10 minutes, until the vegetables are cooked.

Stir in the spinach and cook a further 2-3 minutes so the spinach wilts. Remove from heat, add rosemary and season with freshly ground pepper.

CELERY SOUP (VEGETARIAN & VEGAN)

Serves 2

1 head of celery, chopped

1 sweet potato, peeled and chopped

950 ml filtered water

1 bunch parsley, roughly chopped

Himalayan salt

1 tablespoon of coconut yogurt (if you're happy to eat dairy, replace with natural yogurt)

Instructions

Chop the celery and potato into small chunks.

Add the celery and potato to 950 ml of water and simmer for 20 minutes.

Add the parsley stalks, keeping the leaves for garnish.

When the vegetables are soft, remove from the heat and liquidise with a hand blender.

Season to taste with Himalayan salt and freshly ground pepper.

Add tablespoon of yogurt and then sprinkle over chopped parsley and serve.

CARROT AND GINGER SOUP (VEGETARIAN & VEGAN)

Serves 2

450g carrots, washed and chopped

1 small sweet potato, washed and chopped

700 ml water or vegetable stock

Ginger root

Himalayan salt

1 orange (to squeeze)

handful of chopped Parsley

Instructions

Juice one-third of the carrots.

Boil the remaining carrots and potato in vegetable stock until tender.

Blend in a food processor until smooth.

Grate in ginger to taste.

Add the carrot juice and season with Himalayan salt.

Add a squeeze of orange and garnish with parsley.

CHICKEN, SPRING PEAS AND ASPARAGUS QUINOA

Serves 2

1 cup quinoa

2 cups water

1 tablespoon coconut oil

½ cup finely chopped red onion

½ pound (about ½ bunch) asparagus woody ends snapped off and discarded

Asparagus spears cut into small pieces

2 cloves garlic, finely chopped

1 cup fresh peas or frozen petit pois, thawed

1 cup shredded cooked chicken

1 cup thinly sliced baby spinach leaves

Himalayan Sea or sea salt and freshly ground pepper

Instructions

Rinse quinoa under cold running water and drain.

Combine water and quinoa in a medium saucepan and bring to a boil. Reduce heat to a simmer, cover and cook (15 minutes).

Meanwhile, heat coconut oil in a large non-stick pan, add onion and asparagus.

Cook, stirring often, until asparagus is tender and bright green, 5-7 minutes. Add garlic and peas and continue cooking for another minute.

Stir in chicken and cooked quinoa. Add the spinach and stir until the spinach wilts, 3-5 minutes. Season with Himalayan salt and freshly ground pepper and serve.

TURKEY & GARLIC ROASTED VEGETABLES

Serves 2

2 free range, organic turkey breasts

1 tablespoon coconut oil (or organic butter)

½ small onion

150 ml (1/4 pint) chicken gravy

1 clove of garlic, chopped

2 medium carrots, quartered

1 small courgette, chopped

50g (2oz) snow peas

Himalayan or sea-salt and freshly ground pepper

Instructions

Preheat the oven 200°C/400°F/gas mark 6

Parboil carrots and snow peas for 4-5 minutes.

Meanwhile grease the bottom of a baking tray with 1 tsp of the coconut oil.

Drain vegetables and spread with the garlic and remaining vegetables over the base of the baking dish.

Spread remaining oil over the vegetables and sprinkle with sea salt and black pepper.

Place in the oven and bake for 30 minutes or until brown. Remove dish from the oven to turn vegetables and return the dish to the oven for a further 30 minutes.

Heat ½ tablespoon of coconut oil in a griddle or frying pan

Slice the turkey breasts in half lengthwise and cook for 12-15 minutes turning occasionally.

With five minutes to go throw the onions in with the turkey until golden brown.

Make up 150 ml of chicken gravy and stir in the onions.

Serve the turkey immediately with the roasted vegetables and pour the chicken gravy as preferred.

QUINOA SALAD WITH AVOCADO, TOMATO, PARSLEY & PINE NUTS (VEGETARIAN & VEGAN)

Serves 1

45 g quinoa

1 tsp coconut oil

120 ml water

Handful of fresh parsley finely chopped

1 avocado, peeled, pitted and diced

1 tomato, chopped

Juice of half a grapefruit

10 pine nuts

Instructions

Heat pan with coconut oil, add quinoa and stir for 1-2 minutes.

Add water, bring to a boil, simmer for 15 minutes then remove from heat. Fluff quinoa with a fork and place on serving bowl/dish. Sprinkle the parsley, avocado and tomato over the top of the cooled quinoa. Pour the grapefruit juice over and toss in the pine nuts. Serve.

BUCKWHEAT PATTIES (BALLS) (VEGETARIAN & VEGAN)

1 cup buckwheat

2 cups water

Some yeast-free vegetable stock

1 pinch of Himalayan salt

3 small carrots

1 small onion

1/2 red bell pepper

Fresh parsley / spices to taste

2 tbsp spelt flour or buckwheat flour

2 tbsp oil (cooled pressed extra virgin olive oil)

Instructions

Bring buckwheat, water, vegetable stock and salt to a boil. Cook for 15 minutes until water is gone making sure not to burn it.

Meanwhile, cut onion and bell pepper into small pieces and shred carrots.

Put everything in a bowl. Add the cooked buckwheat and season with spices and flour. Stir. Form 4-6 patties, put olive oil in a pan and roast the patties gently (on both sides) until golden brown.

Tip: Each time you make the patties use different veggies until you find your perfect combination. Serve with a fresh, mixed salad.

ROASTED SPICY PARSNIP (VEGETARIAN & VEGAN)

2 large parsnips, peeled and sliced into chips

1 large onion peeled and quartered (optional)

1 tbsp Coconut oil, melted

2 tsp paprika

½ tsp chili powder

Salt and black pepper

Instructions

Preheat oven to 230C/450F/Gas mark 8

Put all the ingredients into a large bowl and toss until the parsnips and onions are coated in coconut oil. Place in a baking tray and cook for 30-40 minutes, turning halfway until golden.

LIME CHILI STIR FRY (VEGETARIAN & VEGAN)

1 bunch Bok-Choi (or other Asian greens)

1/2 bunch Tuscan kale

3-4 spring onions (scallions)

Handful of Sugar Snap Peas

1/2 packet of beansprouts

8 florets of broccoli (from one head of broccoli)

1/4 cabbage (red or green) finely chopped

1 courgette

1 lime, juiced

2 hot chilli peppers finely chopped

1/2 bunch of coriander

100ml vegetable stock

45g Quinoa

1 generous teaspoon of coconut oil

Instructions

Pulp the coriander with a pestle and mortar along with the finely chopped chilli, adding lime juice as you go to make a dressing/sauce. Then set aside to infuse.

Simmer quinoa (one part quinoa with two parts water) for 15 minutes. While quinoa is cooking, chop all the vegetables into small strips (so that they'll cook reasonably quickly).

To 'fry' the vegetables, I recommend gently heating the coconut oil in a pan and then adding the vegetables, followed by a little of the vegetable stock, so that the steam cooks the veggies. You can add more and more (you may not need all 100ml) until the veggies are cooked, and crunchy still (you don't want them soggy).

Now place all ingredients on a bed of fluffy quinoa and cover with the coriander and lime-chilli sauce.

Serve, piping hot.

CHICKPEA PATTIES WITH TOMATO, CUCUMBER & MINT SALAD (VEGETARIAN & VEGAN)

Serves 2

2 sweet potatoes

1 can of chick peas

2 cloves of garlic, crushed

3 spring onions, sliced

Handful of chopped coriander

1 tablespoon of polenta

1 cucumber

2 tomatoes

1/2 fresh lime, juiced

1 tbsp of pumpkin seeds

1 tbsp of sesame seeds

1/2 cup of soy yoghurt

1 handful of fresh mint

Coconut or olive oil

Instructions

Peel and steam the sweet potato until tender and then mash this with the chickpeas in a bowl. Add the garlic, onion and coriander. Shape this mixture into little patties (burgers) and coat in the polenta. Refrigerate for one hour.

As the hour approaches, turn on the oven to 180 degrees to preheat. While these are cooling, prepare the salad by slicing the cucumber and tomatoes and mixing in a bowl with the seeds, juice and mint. Once combined, stir through the soy yoghurt and season.

Now the patties are cooled, warm a medium pan with a little coconut or olive oil and lightly cook until browned very slightly. Transfer to the oven to cook through and then serve with the salad and dressing.

ROAST CHICKEN – NUT & ONION

1.2Kg – whole chicken

6 tbsp almond butter

5 tbsp olive oil

200ml chicken stock

1 bay leaf

2 tsp dried sage

2 tsp dried rosemary

2 tsp dried parsley

1 tsp paprika

8 shallots, peeled

30ml balsamic vinegar

Himalayan salt and ground black pepper to taste

Instructions

Preheat oven to 200C/425F/Gas mark 7

Combine the herbs and spices (sage through paprika) in a bowl and set aside. Season cavity of chicken with Himalayan salt, pepper and 2 tsp of the herb mix. Place bay leaf inside and tie the legs.

Brush the chicken with olive oil and half the herb mix. Spoon shallots, cover and sprinkle with remaining herb mix. Bake for 1 hour 15 minutes or until the juices run clear. Cover the chicken with tin foil to keep warm.

Pour the juices from the roasting tin into a saucepan and add stock. Bring to a boil and simmer for 5 minutes. Whisk in almond butter. Serve over carved chicken.

STEAMED SALMON & HUMMUS

Serves 1

1 salmon fillet

½ lemon, juice

120 ml filtered water / mineral water

parsley

Instructions

Place fillet skin side down on a dinner plate, place on top of a saucepan of boiling water, add lemon juice and water to surround the salmon. Cover with saucepan lid and cook for 10 – 15 minutes until salmon is cooked through.

Remove salmon onto another serving plate, add one tablespoon of hummus. Eat with a mixed salad or steamed vegetables. Add olive oil and sprinkle fresh parsley over top.

QUINOA & CAJUN CHICKEN

Serves 4

500 G skinless, boneless chicken thighs

1 tbsp Cajun seasoning

100g Quinoa

1 tablespoon coconut oil

600ml hot chicken stock

100g mango, peeled and cut into chunks

1 tbsp olive oil

400g tin chick peas, rinsed and drained

2 red onions, thickly sliced

1 pepper, thickly sliced

1 bunch spring onions, chopped

Small bunch of coriander, finely chopped

Instructions

Rinse quinoa and fry in non-stick pan with a tablespoon of coconut oil for a couple of minutes, until it smells a little nutty.

Meanwhile cut chicken thighs into bite-sized pieces and toss through Cajun seasoning. Place chicken in a baking dish and cook in oven on 180c (160 fan), 350f, gas mark 4 for 20-25 minutes. You may need to stir occasionally.

In a large saucepan, cook quinoa over a high heat in the chicken stock for 15 mins. Stir occasionally to avoid sticking to the bottom.

In a large non-stick frying pan, stir-fry the red onions, spring onions and pepper over a high heat in olive oil until soft. Approximately 5 minutes. You may want to add small splashes of water if the stir fry dries out and starts to stick.

Add chickpeas and mango to the quinoa. Stir in, lower heat and continue to cook for 2-3 mins. Then stir in onions and pepper mixture. Cook for a further 1-2 minutes.

Stir in half the chopped coriander and spoon the Cajun chicken quinoa into a serving dish. Sprinkle over the remaining coriander and serve immediately.

Tip: For a spicier dish, use an extra tbsp. of Cajun spices or add some fresh chopped chillies when cooking the onions and pepper.

CRAB STEW

Serves 1

50 g tomatoes, diced

2 garlic cloves, minced

100ml fish stock

1 orange, juiced

1 tsp oregano

¼ tsp cayenne pepper

½ lime, fresh chopped

200g crab meat

Instructions

In a large saucepan combine tomatoes, garlic, stock, orange juice, oregano, cayenne pepper and bring to a simmer over medium heat.

Reduce heat to low and simmer for 5 minutes until sauce thickens. Stir in lime and crab meat. Cook another 5 minutes. Serve.

COURGETTE HUMMUS (VEGETARIAN & VEGAN)

Serves 4

2 courgettes, peeled & chopped

1 lemon, juiced

3 garlic cloves, minced

50 g tahini

1 tsp cumin

1 tsp smoked paprika

3 tbsp olive oil

Himalayan salt and ground black pepper to taste

Instructions

Place all the ingredients in a high-powered blender, blend until smooth and thick. You may need to add a little filtered water.

Divide the hummus between 4 ramekins and chill in the fridge.

Serve with raw crudités (slices of carrot, celery, peppers, broccoli heads).

GRILLED/GRIDDLED CHINESE CHICKEN

Serves 1

1 chicken breast, butterfly cut

1 corn on the cob

1 red pepper

1 bag of mixed salad leaves

2 tsp organic honey

1 tsp olive oil

1 tbsp coconut oil

1 tbsp Chinese five spice

1 tsp soy sauce

Instructions

In a small bowl mix 1 tsp of honey with Chinese five spice and soy sauce. Brush this marinade onto a butterfly chicken breast (cut through the width).

Heat griddle on medium flame with 1 tbsp coconut oil. Place corn on the cob onto the griddle. Turn every three minutes. After 10 minutes the cob should be deep gold in colour. Remove from the griddle and allow to cool.

Meanwhile place chicken breast on the griddle. Depending on thickness of the breast, it should cook through after 4-5 minutes on each side.

Dice red pepper. Remove corn kernels with a sharp knife. Chop cooked chicken into small chunks.

Make salad dressing by mixing the olive oil with 1 tsp of honey.

Dress salad leaves with the honey/oil dressing. Toss in chicken, sweet corn and red pepper.

Serve and eat or add to plastic container for lunch box idea.

COD CEVICHE

Serves 2

450 g cod fillets without skin

Juice of 1 orange

Juice of 6 limes

Small red onion, thinly sliced

30 g fresh coriander, stalks removed

1 red chilli, deseeded and sliced

Pinch of Himalayan salt

Optional, garnish with lime wedges

Instructions

Cut fish into 1 cm cubes. Put in a glass bowl and sprinkle with salt. Set aside for 20 minutes. Add orange juice and 90% of the lime juice. Submerge the fish. Cover & chill in the fridge for 2 hours.

Mix the onion with the remaining lime juice.

Use a slotted spoon and serve the fish into a ceramic serving bowl. Drain the onion. Lightly toss the fish with onion, chillies and fresh coriander. Serve with a green salad and, if desired, fresh lime quarters.

BEAN SPROUT & RED CABBAGE SALAD (VEGETARIAN & VEGAN)

Serves 2

50 g green cabbage, shredded

50 g red cabbage, shredded

2 spring onions, chopped

3 raw brussell sprouts, thinly sliced

1 medium carrot, grated

25g bean sprouts

25g raisins

25g cashews, chopped

1 tbsp sesame seeds

Dressing

2 tbsp olive oil

1 tbsp sesame oil

1 tbsp apple cider vinegar

1 tsp tamari

2 tsp honey

1 tsp fresh ginger, grated

Instructions

Place all the dressing ingredients into a small bowl and whisk together.

In a large bowl toss the dressing with the salad ingredients, except cashews and sesame seeds, until well coated.

Sprinkle on cashews and sesame seeds and serve.

WARM CHICKEN SALAD

Serves 1

150 g cooked chicken breast, diced

½ apple, diced

1 spring onion, sliced

10 g chopped walnuts

30 g celery, chopped

2 Kos lettuce leaves, shredded

¼ cucumber, diced

¾ tbsp balsamic vinegar

1 tbsp olive oil

Instructions

In a small bowl mix together the balsamic vinegar and olive oil.

In a large bowl toss together all the ingredients with the salad dressing.

SPICY VEGGIE BURGERS (VEGETARIAN)

Serves 2

1 small onion, diced

zest of 1 lemon

410 g tinned chick peas, drained

31 g fresh coriander

1 tsp harissa

1 small egg, beaten

1 tbsp olive oil

Instructions

Place all the ingredients except the egg and oil into a food processor and mix. Slowly add egg until the mixture starts to bind. You won't need to use all the egg.

Form the mix into 4 burgers and chill in the fridge for 2 hours or more.

Brush each burger with a little oil before grilling. Grill for 5 mins each side.

Serve with seasonal vegetable or green salad.

SALAD NICOISE

Serves 2

Small tin of tuna, drained

50 g green beans, topped, tailed and steamed

1 hard-boiled egg, quartered

8 black olives, halved

2 chopped anchovy fillets

1 tbsp olive oil

1 tsp lemon juice

1 tsp Dijon mustard

Instructions

Mix Olive oil, lemon juice and mustard together. Add to remaining ingredients in salad bowl.

SCALLOPS

Serves 2

750 g scallops

30 g coconut flour

30 ml coconut or olive oil 1 tbsp fresh parsley, chopped

1 tsp garlic, minced

1 tsp ground peppercorns

1 lemon

Generous splash of white wine

Instructions

In a large non-stick pan, heat 20 ml of oil on high heat. Add the scallops and lower the heat to medium.

Slightly brown one side of the scallops before turning and browning the other side. This takes 3-4 mins in total. Add the remaining olive oil, garlic and parsley. Sauté and toss the scallops for 2 more minutes.

Add the white wine and cook one more minute. Serve scallops immediately with lemon wedges.

FISH POTATO BAKE

Serves 4

375 g sweet potato, peeled & cubed

145g salmon fillet

122g tinned tuna, drained

2 eggs

Instructions

Preheat oven to 180c (160 fan), 350f, Gas Mark 4.

In a small saucepan, boil sweet potatoes in water until soft, about 10 minutes. Drain.

Put all the ingredients into a food processor and blend until smooth.

Pour contents into a silicon loaf pan & bake for 20-25 minutes until firm throughout.

Serve immediately with green vegetables or salad.

BEETROOT SALAD (VEGETARIAN & VEGAN)

Serves 2

1-2 raw beetroots, grated

4 spring onions, sliced

1 red chilli, deseeded & chopped

1 tbsp olive oil

1 tbsp lime juice

1 tbsp fresh mint, chopped

Instructions

In a small bowl whisk together the olive oil, lime juice, mint and dash of organic balsamic vinegar.

Place remaining ingredients in a large bowl and toss together with dressing.

Serve.

PRAWN HOTPOT

Serves 4

375 g cooked prawns, peeled

375 g smoked salmon, diced

250 g tin chopped tomatoes

1 onion, chopped

1 pepper, chopped

1 tsp smoked paprika

2 tbsp coconut oil

3 celery stalks, chopped

2 garlic cloves, crushed

1 tsp dried chilli Flakes

300g cauliflower, grated

Instructions

Heat oil in large saucepan. Add ham and onions and fry over low heat for 1-2 minutes. Next add pepper, garlic and celery and cook for a further minute.

Drain juice from tomatoes and add them to saucepan along with paprika & chilli. Stir in prawns. Cover pan and cook for 10 minutes. Check to be sure there's enough liquid, if not add splashes of water.

Add grated cauliflower. Stir and mix well. Allow to cook/warm through for 2 minutes.

Serve immediately.

GRIDDLED AUBERGINE (VEGETARIAN & VEGAN)

Serves 6

2 aubergines, sliced vertically

2 tbsp olive oil

250 g coconut yogurt

3 tbsp almond butter

1 garlic clove, crushed

Juice of one lemon

2 tbsp coriander, chopped

2 tbsp parsley, chopped

2 tbsp mint, chopped

Instructions

Brush each aubergine slice with some oil and place slices on griddle. Cook for 2-3 mins on each side until golden brown and tender.

Mix the yogurt with the almond butter, garlic, lemon juice and herbs. Top the aubergines with yogurt dressing.

AVOCADO & TOFU DIP (VEGETARIAN & VEGAN)

Serves 1 - 2

1 avocado

1/2 package of silken tofu

1 large tomato

1 clove of garlic

1 small onion (try brown or red)

Some fresh parsley (if available, but not vital)

Freshly ground black pepper and Himalayan/sea salt

Instructions

Peel and core the avocado, roughly chop the tofu, tomato, garlic and onion, rip up the parsley and throw it all in a blender and blend until smooth!

If you want to thin it out a little you can add a little olive oil and some filtered water until you get the consistency you like.

Serve with crudité.

SALMON ASPARAGUS PARCELS

Serves 1

1 packet of asparagus spears

125 g smoked salmon

1 lemon, quartered

Black pepper to taste

Instructions

Lightly steam asparagus for 1-2 minutes so they still have crunch/bite left.

Wrap bundles of spears with smoked salmon slices. Squeeze over lemon juice and grind over black pepper to taste.

SPICY TUNA IN TOMATO SAUCE

Serves 2

2 tuna steaks (100 g each)

1 tablespoon coconut oil plus extra for brushing tuna

2 shallots, peeled and chopped

½ teaspoon smoked paprika

¼ teaspoon chilli powder (add more if you like it stronger)

1 x 200g (7oz) can chopped tomatoes

1 teaspoon tomato puree

1 clove garlic, crushed

Juice of half an orange

1 teaspoon balsamic vinegar

Instructions

Sauce: Heat a tablespoon of olive oil in a small saucepan over medium heat. Add the shallots and let them soften for a few minutes. Add paprika and chilli powder and stir. Add the tomatoes, tomato puree and garlic, stir well and bring to a simmering point. Stir in the orange juice and vinegar and simmer gently for 5 minutes to blend flavours.

Tuna: Brush each steak with a tablespoon of coconut oil and cover with a good grinding of black pepper. Wrap each steak tightly in foil. Heat a pan until hot, put the wrapped tuna in the pan and press down hard to cook it. Turnover and repeat This takes about 5 minutes on each side. Unwrap and serve with sauce and a large, fresh green salad. Sprinkle over fresh herbs of your choice.

DRESSINGS

Homemade healthy ways of dressing your food

CHILLI LIME DRESSING (VEGETARIAN & VEGAN)

1 long red chilli, deseeded, finely chopped

Juice of 1 lime

1 cup / 240ml, cold pressed extra virgin olive oil

Instructions

Place all the ingredients into a sterilized glass jar and shake vigorously. Add Himalayan sea salt and black pepper to taste. Can be stored in the fridge for a few days. Add to salads. Add to quinoa, vegetable and meat dishes or fish with salad dishes etc.

CITRUS DRESSING (VEGETARIAN & VEGAN)

1/3 cup fresh lemon and/or lime juice

3/4 cup cold pressed extra virgin olive oil

1 tablespoon flax seed oil

1 clove garlic, chopped finely

½ tsp ground oregano

¼ tsp dried rosemary

1 tsp dried basil

½ tsp ground cumin

Pinch Himalayan salt

Pinch cayenne pepper

Instructions

Place all the ingredients into a blender, mix well. Serve and store in a sterilised glass jar. Can be stored in the fridge for a few days. Add to salads, stir-fry and cooked meals, after cooking.

THOUSAND ISLAND DRESSING

100 g cashews

6 sundried tomatoes

3 tbsp lemon juice

1 tsp English mustard

1 celery stalk, finely diced

¼ red onion, finely diced

Instructions

Soak the cashews in water for 4 hours and drain. Soak the sundried tomatoes until soft and drain.

Blend all ingredients together, except onion and celery. You may need to add more water. Once smooth, transfer to a bowl and mix in celery and onion.

Let dressing rest overnight in a sealed jar before serving. Can be stored in the fridge for a few days.

HOMEMADE MAYONNAISE

1 free range egg

1 tablespoon cider vinegar

300 ml extra virgin cold press olive oil

Pinch of dried tarragon

Instructions

Break egg into blender, add the tarragon and blend for 30 seconds.

Add the cider vinegar and blend.

Keep blender running, whilst adding a slow, steady stream of oil. The sauce should start to thicken after half the oil has been added.

Continue to pour the oil until entire mixture has combined. Serve.

Transfer to sterile jar with lid and store in the fridge.

BALSAMIC MARINADE (VEGETARIAN & VEGAN)

¼ cup balsamic vinegar

¼ cup olive oil

1 rosemary prig, finely chopped

Instructions

Whisk ingredients together in small mixing bowl.

Pour over chosen meat or fish and cover.

Marinate in the fridge for 4 hours.

Reference

YOUR BEST BODY FUEL – BALANCED MEALS

Aim for natural, whole, unprocessed and ideally organic foods. If the food you're eating wasn't plucked from the ground, picked from a tree or running around freely and in its most natural form, then it's processed.

The five components of your best body fuel

1. Best Carbs – Carbohydrates
2. Best Protein
3. Best Fats
4. Water (2.5 litres per day)
5. Best Portion size

What are (Carbs) Carbohydrates?

There are two types of carbohydrates

1. Complex carbs (containing fibre and starch)
2. Simple carbs (sugar)

Where are carbohydrates found?

Fruit, vegetables, grains, milk and any food containing sugar.

Why do we need carbohydrates?

To make glucose (sugar) for energy

What is protein?

There are two types of protein

1. Animal protein

2. Plant protein

Protein contains 20 amino acids, nine of which are essential to the body. Plant protein may not contain all essential amino acids.

Where is protein found?

Animal protein is found in meat, fish, poultry, dairy and eggs. Plant protein is found in pulses, grains such as quinoa, soy and nuts.

Why do we need protein?

The body needs protein for proper growth and functioning. Protein comprises the building blocks of cells and helps maintain muscles, tendons and ligaments.

What is fat?

There are three types of fat

1. Saturated – solid at cold room temperature such as butter and coconut oil

2. Monounsaturated – liquid at room temperature but will start to solidify in the fridge, such as olive oil

3. Polyunsaturated – liquid both at room temperature and in the fridge such as sunflower oil. Omega 3, 6 and 9.

Why do we need fats?

Fat is very needed in the body. Omega 3 and 6 are vital in proper brain function. In addition, fat:

- Aids absorption of fat-soluble vitamins such as a, d, e and k
- Regulates immune system and hormone production
- Supports cell growth and protects your organs
- Keeps your body warm and is a fuel source at low levels of intense exercise
- Increases oxygen rate, metabolic rate, energy levels and stamina
- Improves mood and concentration
- Helps to slow the rate of sugar released into the blood stream
- Provides energy at low level energy exercise level

SHOPPING LIST

I've compiled this list to provide you with foods for sensible, healthy eating, and to ensure you're giving your body what it needs.

Store Cupboard

CEREALS AND GRAINS: Porridge oats (ideally gluten free), quinoa, brown rice, buckwheat pasta and brown rice pasta

DRIED FRUIT: Figs, prunes, dates and apricots (unsulphured)

SEEDS: Sesame seeds, pumpkin seeds, sunflower seeds and golden and Brown linseed.

NUTS: Raw almonds, Brazil and walnuts

SPICES & SEASONING: Nutmeg, curry, paprika, cinnamon, bay leaves, cumin, coriander, Himalayan salt, whole black peppercorns and organic vegetable stock cubes

OILS: Extra virgin organic raw coconut oil, extra virgin cold pressed olive oil and organic flaxseed oil

SAUCES: Organic balsamic vinegar, organic soya sauce and organic apple cider vinegar

WHEAT FLOUR ALTERNATIVES: Coconut flour, rice flour and almond flour

PULSES: Chick peas, butter beans, lentils (red, green, brown), red kidney beans and hummus

DRINKS: Herbal tea such as mint, rooibos, chamomile, ginger, peppermint and curcumin. Still mineral water and pressed or squeezed fresh fruit juices (dilute to ½ water and ½ juice)

NATURAL SWEETENERS: Agave nectar, organic honey and stevia

Fresh Basics (use within 7 days)

FRESH HERBS: Parsley, rosemary, sage, thyme, basil, mint and coriander

VEGETABLES, FRUITS AND ROOTS: Ginger root, sweet potatoes, celery, broccoli, onions, garlic, courgettes, leeks, carrots, lemons, parsnips, green salad, tomatoes and red onion

DAIRY

Free range eggs

Organic unsalted butter

Plain natural bio cow milk yogurt

Plain natural bio goat milk yogurt

Goat cheese

Cottage cheese

Feta cheese

NON DAIRY MILK PRODUCTS

Almond milk

Soya milk

BREAD & IDEAL ALTERNATIVES

Organic oat cakes

Pumpernickel bread

Rye bread (okay if gluten tolerant)

Grain bread (wheat free, gluten free and yeast free)

HEALTHY SNACK IDEAS

- 1 apple, plus 2-3 almonds or a dessert spoon of pumpkin seeds

- Organic oat cakes (with a topping such as raw organic almond butter or hummus or avocado)

- Organic hummus with crudités such as slices of carrots, cucumber, peppers, celery or tomato. Dip ½ tub of hummus maximum.

- Half an avocado with: olive oil, apple cider vinegar, squeeze of fresh lemon juice, Himalayan salt & pepper and eat out with a spoon.

Tip: Aim to achieve your balance of best fats, best carbs and best proteins for every meal,

If you need to snack to achieve your balanced mini-meal aim to eat nuts and seeds with fruit.

Gratitude

Write your five things to be grateful for every day, ideally first thing in the morning. Write your gratitude list in the present tense even if it's in the future and not yet manifested. Always begin your sentence with *I am so happy and grateful for…*

Imagine you have it and are living it right now. Be grateful for the good in your life and the good that's on its way.

CREATE YOUR OWN GRATITUDE LIST

Use those that resonate with you below:

I am so happy and grateful for my amazing health.

I am so happy and grateful for feeling so bright and alive with such boundless energy.

I am so happy and grateful for feeling healthy and vibrant all the time.

I am so happy and grateful that I wake feeling rested and refreshed after a good night's sleep.

I am so happy and grateful it comes naturally to me to see the good in people.

I am so happy and grateful for being so in tune with my body and giving it what it needs.

I am so happy and grateful for the promotion at work and that my career is taking off.

I am so happy and grateful for living in such a friendly, kind neighborhood.

I am so happy and grateful for such a fulfilling job with such supportive colleagues.

I am so happy and grateful for my ability to learn new skills every day and be an expert in my field.

I am so happy and grateful for being a kind, giving and loving person and that the people attracted into my life are also kind, giving and loving.

www.annascanlan.com

I am so happy and grateful for my positive contribution to the world.

I am so happy and grateful for being appreciated at work, at home and by everyone I come into contact with.

I am so happy and grateful that the right person always shows up.

I am so happy and grateful for such a happy, healthy, love-rich family.

I am so happy and grateful for such a loving, calm and joyful family.

I am so happy and grateful for so much love in my life.

I am so happy and grateful for the love of my life and that we are the pure definition of soul mates.

I am happy for my tidy, peaceful and loving home.

I am so happy and grateful for the fun in my life and the regular belly laughs.

I am so happy and grateful for my loving, loyal best friend soul mate.

I am so happy and grateful for the money flowing into my bank account easily.

I am so happy and grateful now that I am able to pay all my bills easily.

I am so happy and grateful for being such a confident person.

I am so happy and grateful for my excellent posture and confident state.

I am so happy and grateful for the great friendships in my life and the great friend that I am.

I am so happy and grateful for my slim, strong body and perfect body.

I am so happy and grateful for being such a positive person, attracting positive people in my life.

I am so happy and grateful for the self-discipline to look after myself for the best life ever.

I am so happy and grateful for my beautiful beachside property.

I am so happy and grateful for the great teachers in my life and for learning subjects I'm so passionate about.

I am so happy and grateful for my life going in the direction of all my wants, desires and dreams.

I am so happy and grateful to look after my physical and mental fitness every day.

I am so happy and grateful for being the best version of me every day.

I am so happy and grateful for my abundant life.

I am so happy and grateful for giving and receiving love easily.

I am so happy for being in such great physical condition.

I am so happy and grateful for clear, positive thinking.

I am so happy and grateful now that I am living this abundant life.

I am so happy and grateful for living in the now and appreciating nature.

I am so happy and grateful for all the creative ideas that come flooding in, especially when I'm taking a shower!

I am so happy and grateful for my playful approach to life and that others find me fun to be around.

About the Author

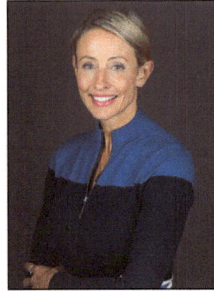

Anna Scanlan is a British woman of 50 years! Half a century young! Anna is vibrant, healthy, energetic and feeling like she's in her 20s! She's always been fascinated by finding natural ways to look and feel young and discovering ways to live longer, live well and enjoy a more purposeful life.

Ms. Scanlan is the author and creator of online transformative programmes. She's a motivator and a little ray of sunshine to inspire others to take charge of their health, fitness and happiness for a brilliant life. She sets a shining example by living the best way, every day.

Anna is an entrepreneur, a highly successful, transformative coaching professional and personal trainer to the every day star. She incorporates holistic solution expertise within fitness, mindset and nutrition strategy. Anna holds a sports science diploma and is qualified in advanced nutrition for weight loss management. Well qualified Personal Trainer and Nutritional Advisor. Bob Proctor Coaching and Mary Morrissey's Dream Builder Coaching. Previously a ski instructor and trampoline coach, Anna is. overflowing with positivity bringing the best out of countless people and successfully achieving the results they seek.

Ms. Scanlan takes immense pride in delivering a top level, red carpet service. She's always looking for ways to serve better, improve and captivate. Coming from a family of school teachers, professors, sports masters and a golf pro, it's in her DNA to teach, share knowledge and get a poignant point across in an understandable and captivating way. She's a brilliant encourager, and instiller of confidence and self-belief. Anna has strong family values and enjoys spending time with dear family.

Anna just simply loves the world and the people in it. She wants to touch the lives of millions of people and imagines a world where everyone is fitter, happier and healthier. She wants to make looking after yourself easy. The 'go to' daily practice. Anna believes life should be a joy and we have the resilience to come back stronger if a low point should show up.

Anna has heavily invested and continues to invest in her physical and mental fitness. She has a burning desire and passion to be the best version of herself to help others better. She's worked out her life purpose and set ambitious goals. Every day she enhances, advances and evolves in the right direction. An eternal student of life. Working on yourself, learning and improving every day.

Anna loves being outside, close to nature and seeing the natural wonders of the world. She thrives in the fresh air, beautiful skies, the stars and being close to our natural environment. She loves feeling calm and tranquil with beautiful landscapes, nature scenes and appreciating the many wonderful creatures we share living on this magical planet.

"I believe we're the best we can be when we help each other. I want to grow a health, fitness and happiness movement of 'likeminded' people who encourage one another to stay on track. The best healthy way. I believe it's possible to re-programme yourself to make positive lasting changes. Added to that, I believe working together will massively increase your chances of success."

I hope you've enjoyed and found this little foundation book, with its five point plan helpful in improving your life quality.

If you're looking to honour and look after your magnificent body and mind some more check out **www.annascanlan.com**

If you haven't already visited yourbestbodyever.com to access the additional components that accompany this book, scan this QR code to go there now.

Your access membership will give you access to the Best Body 5 components of fitness video workouts and your daily grading accomplishment document.

You'll also receive Peak Living Secrets, Tips, Motivators and Special Offers to help make the most of yourself and make the most of your special life.

Best Ever program range and complemented programs with experts incorporating the entire best life ever solutions. Incorporating great health, fitness, wellness, nutrition, lifestyle, confidence and mindset. The full spectrum of physical and mental fitness and greater life coaching.

Best Ever program range and complemented programs with experts incorporating the entire best life ever solution. Programs coming soon. Soon to be available:

- Best Ever Morning routine
- Best Ever Life Coach
- Best Ever Happy Hormones
- Best Ever HIIT for MAX Weight loss
- Best Ever Motivators
- Best Body 5 Components of Fitness
- Best Ever Gratitude
- Best Ever mind
- Best Ever Body Sculpture
- Best Ever Kitchen Food Makeover

- Best Ever Buddies
- Best Ever Flat Tummy
- Best Ever Restaurant meal choice
- Best Ever Quick Meals

All programmes are geared up to provide forever solutions that are holistic, nourishing and give your body and mind what they need. The programs instil daily practice, daily habits and encourage a lifestyle of long-term great health, happiness and fitness. A natural approach. As you work through the programs you'll find at least one point per program that resonates with you, evolves you and your healthy lifestyle and stays with you for the rest of your life.

You may have realized by now that diets, fads and quick fixes don't work. They set you up to fail from the start as you rely on will power alone (which runs out pretty quickly) and sets your focus on what you're missing out on.

Your Best Ever programs have been designed for busy people in a straight forward manner. You'll be clear about what you're being asked to do, how it serves you and how it's effective and worthwhile.

All programs are on point and made really easy to understand to encourage you to stick with it.

Imagine living in a body that is fit and healthy. How much more you could do? How would you feel?

Imagine if you trained your thinking mind. How much more joy do you think you'd experience? What would your life look and feel like?

We're only on this phenomenal planet for such a short time, why not enjoy your life even more with your amazing body and thinking mind? You can do it. I can help.

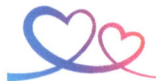

Hearts to be HEARD

Giving a Voice to Creativity!

Wouldn't you love to help the physically, spiritually, and mentally challenged?

Would you like to make a difference in a child's life?

Imagine giving them:
confidence; self-esteem; pride; and self-respect.
Perhaps a legacy that lives on.

You see, that's what we do.
We give a voice to the creativity in their hearts,
for those who would otherwise not be heard.

Join us by going to

HeartstobeHeard.com

Help us, help others.

www.ingramcontent.com/pod-product-compliance
Lightning Source LLC
Chambersburg PA
CBHW060804270326
41927CB00002B/45